'The language the authors use is exemplary of solution focused work: loud and clear, no nonsense. I particularly like the reflective parts, with the kinds of questions a solution focused worker would ask their client. A book you should have in your library!'

— Els Mattelin, therapist and co-author of
Autism and Solution-focused Practice

Using Solution Focused Practice with Adults in Health and Social Care

Judith Milner and Steve Myers

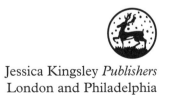

Jessica Kingsley *Publishers*
London and Philadelphia

First published in 2017
by Jessica Kingsley Publishers
73 Collier Street
London N1 9BE, UK
and
400 Market Street, Suite 400
Philadelphia, PA 19106, USA

www.jkp.com

Library of Congress Cataloging in Publication Data
Names: Milner, Judith, 1941- author. | Myers, Steve (John Stephen), 1959-
    author.
Title: Using solution focused practice with adults in health and social care
    / Judith Milner and Steve Myers.
Description: London ; Philadelphia : Jessica Kingsley Publishers, 2017.
Identifiers: LCCN 2017022505| ISBN 9781785920677 (alk. paper) | ISBN
    9781784503253 (E-ISBN)
Subjects: | MESH: Counseling--methods | Adult | Interview,
    Psychological--methods | Professional-Patient Relations | Social Work
Classification: LCC RC480 | NLM WM 55 | DDC
616.89/1--dc23 LC record available at
https://lccn.loc.gov/2017022505

British Library Cataloguing in Publication Data
A CIP catalogue record for this book is available from the British Library

ISBN 978 1 78592 067 7
eISBN 978 1 78450 325 3

Printed and bound in Great Britain

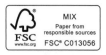

To Alasdair Macdonald for his intellectual rigour, unstinting personal encouragement and leading role in the development of solution focused practice.

Contents

Chapter One

Useful Conversations

Positive Approaches to Working with Adults

In writing this book, we have endeavoured to highlight how solution focused practice can be useful to a broad range of practitioners working with adults – whether in health and social care, with older age and end of life care, with physical or intellectual disability and mental ill-health. These can be nurses, health visitors, occupational therapists, physiotherapists, social carers, social workers, housing support workers and counsellors in residential or community-based settings. We aim to offer a unifying theoretical underpinning which outlines the basic philosophy of the approach and what it looks like in reality.

The techniques described in this book are compatible with the professional requirements of all those professions listed above, and they can be used to help promote the 'Well-being' principle of the Care Act 2014 (in England) in the areas of: personal dignity; physical and mental health and emotional well-being; protection from abuse and neglect; control by the individual over their day-to-day life; domestic, family and personal; suitability of living accommodation; participation in work, education, training or recreation; social and economic well-being and the individual's contribution to society.

They also help to meet the principle outlined in the Social Services and Well-being (Wales) Act 2014, which specifies that 'People have control over what support they need, making decisions about their care and support as an equal partner' (p.3) even where a person appears to be very muddled in their thinking, as the following example shows.

CASE EXAMPLE

Mrs Brown was perhaps a little too decisive about giving up her own home for residential care. When seen at her bedside in hospital, where she had been admitted after a fall, she had difficulty remembering where she lived, where she was currently and who had been to see her. For example, when Judith asked if she could sit on her bed while they talked, she was unsure whose bed it was. Although some of her memories were dim, the gaps did not divide easily into long- or short-term ones and it was possible that her confusion was exacerbated by a long period of self-neglect when she had refused help, and perhaps some underlying sadness as she made several comments about having lived long enough.

The different components of her confusion included forgetfulness, muddle, sadness and, possibly, weariness resulting from a prehospital period of struggle and difficulty with everyday living. Solution focused questions were asked to get a feel of how this seemingly confused elderly person saw herself and whether her perception matched the presentation of herself to both ward and multi-disciplinary team members.

After several conversations with Mrs Brown in hospital, it emerged that she wanted a residential placement where she would not have to worry about cooking and managing money. What continued to be important to her was the type and location of the residential home, which she hoped would be lively, with friendly residents, and near enough to her old home so that she could resume social activities at her church as soon as her mobility improved and her pain eased. Pain, she said, caused her to worry more and this had probably prevented her from maintaining her links with the community in which she had lived most of her life and which centred on her local church.

A visit was arranged so that Mrs Brown could spend some time in a home selected as most meeting her hopes. She became much more animated and less muddled as she left hospital and recognised familiar surroundings; even her mobility improved and it was easier to get her out of the wheelchair at the home than it had been to get her into it in hospital.

The visit proved tiring for Mrs Brown, who greeted Judith on arrival to collect her with a heartfelt, 'Oh, I am glad you've come. I know you, don't I? I don't know where I am.' She was much more muddled on the return journey, which took her past her old home; she thought someone else was living there, she had forgotten which of her first two names her husband called her by, and she was unsure why she was going back to hospital – although she was keen to get to bed.

Talking with her the next day when she was rested, she gave a coherent account of chatting with some women she didn't know about having their hair done and, at first, she seemed to be talking about old memories. She then said, 'I don't think I know them… But if they can have their hair done, it must be a nice place. I'll be all right there. I can't remember their names… But they were friendly.' When well enough, she was admitted to the home and settled in easily; she remained muddled about many things but had her hair permed immediately and was clearly enjoying the company of the other residents.

While specific training requirements in different sectors will inevitably differ, one unifying theme running through all sectors is the importance of hearing the voice of the person. Traditionally, our knowledge of people and accepted ways of working with them has been influenced by psychiatric and psychological knowledge. This is extremely useful, but it is fundamentally problem-based, with people categorised so that they can be more easily understood and 'treated' by expert professionals.

It can be argued that categorisation is helpful; for example, an adult diagnosed with attention deficit hyperactivity disorder (ADHD) will then receive the medical intervention (medication, therapy) that is considered required, and the diagnosis provides an understanding of why they are behaving in a particular way. An alternative argument, however, is that this diagnosis then places the 'problem' within the person, which can lead to the person becoming pathologised: 'labels help us recognise patterns of behaviour but should not be mistaken for people doing that behaviour' (Winbolt 2011, p.72).

Furthermore, categorisation can define and conclude what intervention is best for the individual without considering their own unique ideas and strengths with regards to what would work best for them in the future:

> we noticed that social workers, parents and partners of people with autism are often concerned that people with autism may be socially isolated because they appear to have few friends. If, however, somebody with autism feels perfectly happy with just one close friend and a few contacts on social media, who are we to judge that this cannot be sufficient for a good and meaningful life? (Mattelin and Volckaert 2017, p.14)

Speech and language therapist, Kidge Burns similarly comments that recovery from incapacitating illness is more likely to be the development of a desired lifestyle rather than simply symptom removal (2016, p.20), whilst psychiatrist Alasdair Macdonald (2011) noted that while many people want to alleviate distressing symptoms of severe mental illness, others prefer to work on life skills, or how to effect an early discharge form hospital.

PRACTICE ACTIVITY

Ahktar was diagnosed as being on the Autistic Spectrum at secondary school and was allocated a support worker to assist him in coping with the other students' boisterous behaviour.

- What are the benefits for Ahktar of his diagnosis?
- What are the possible negative impacts for Ahktar of his diagnosis?
- How can you make best use of the benefits of the labels given to the people with whom you work?
- How can you use these benefits whilst avoiding any negative impacts?

Whatever your profession, the best ways of working with people are those in which workers practise collaboratively as respected partners in an agreed activity. This approach is applicable to all workforce contexts, including community and residential, social and health. Additionally, it needs to be applied whether you are working with individuals, their families or groups, able-bodied or disabled, and whatever their intellectual ability. There are a number of ways of working with people that fulfil all these criteria. For example, narrative approaches have been used in work with whole communities at high risk of diabetes, as well as small groups with anorexia (Epston 1998), and the strengths model recognises and values resilience and resourcefulness (Edwards and Pedrotti 2004; Saleebey 2013). Another approach is focusing on solutions (Berg and Steiner 2003; Milner 2001; Milner and Myers 2016; Myers 2008) – the focus of this book.

Although narrative and strengths perspectives influence our work, we choose to concentrate on solution focused practice. This method was developed from asking people what worked best for them, and keeping all these elements and discarding any others (de Shazer 1988, 1994). Solution focused practice aims to restore people's problem-solving potential and mobilise their own inner resources or resourcefulness. This we believe to be an appropriate and effective unifying theory and practice for all branches of the adult's workforce. For example, studies in Europe, Japan and China show solution focused practice to be an effective way of increasing medication compliance and improved communication between patients and health care professionals (Cui *et al.* 2008; Macdonald 2011; Mishima 2012; Panayotov, Strahilov and Anichkina 2012).

Solution focused practice

A major reason why we promote this way of working is because a central element is being aware of how we talk and listen to people. Talking is not a neutral activity; how we talk about events and ourselves has the capacity to change how we are: 'Finding a name for something is a way of conjuring it into existence, or making it possible for people to see a pattern where they didn't see one before' (Rheingold 1998, cited in Elgin 2000, p.57). Thus, how we describe or talk about things, whether these are experiences in general or our interactions with others, provides a specific understanding. Consider the words that you may have heard exchanged between professionals about people in both informal and formal settings. On occasions when the descriptions have been pathologising of an individual, how helpful are these when attempting to move people beyond their problems? If you imagine having a supervisor who constantly focused on things that were not going well in your practice or was critical of your work and never acknowledged your skills and strengths, how would that affect you? The importance is in achieving a balanced perspective so that concerns are not minimised alongside locating people's abilities and qualities to support them in moving forward.

PRACTICE ACTIVITY

- Go online and find the DSM–5.

    - Choose one or two mental illness diagnoses listed in the DSM–5; for example, borderline personality disorder,

> dependent personality disorder, attention deficit hyper-activity disorder or social anxiety disorder.

- Look at the behaviour criteria for these diagnoses.

    - See if you actually have the potential to be diagnosed with any such disorder.

- In what other way could you describe these behaviours?

- Choose one or two diagnoses listed in the DSM–5; for example, borderline personality disorder, dependent personality disorder, attention deficit hyperactivity disorder or social anxiety disorder.

- Look at the criteria for these diagnoses and see if you actually have the potential to be diagnosed with any such disorder.

- In what other way could you describe these behaviours?

Thompson (2003) says that we cannot expect to be successful in our attempts to communicate if we are not able to listen effectively. We examine effective listening more fully in the next chapter but, here, we briefly mention some barriers to effective listening that a problem focus may inadvertently encourage:

- A person may have many features of a recognised problem, such as Parkinson's disease or dyslexia, but this does not mean that the person is like *all* people with Parkinson's disease or dyslexia.

- Categorising people has the advantage of making them eligible for extra resources, but it can have the disadvantage of leading you to assume that you know what the problem is and indulging in mind reading.

- Similarly, thinking you know what problem you are dealing with sometimes means that you only listen to the bits you want to hear and then you may filter out much of what the person is saying.

- Equally, being certain that we know what the problem is, and de facto, the solution, means we stop listening.

- Funnily enough, offering advice to people on how to solve their problems closes down effective listening.

PRACTICE ACTIVITY

The next time someone consults you about a problem (this can be a friend, colleague or person with whom you are working):

- Think what advice you are going to offer but *don't do this yet.*

- Ask them what they have tried so far, what worked and what didn't.

- If something worked a little bit, talk with them about how they can do more of it.

- If nothing worked, ask them what they could do differently.

- Ask if they have any resources for this.

- Discover what resources outside of themselves they need.

- If it hasn't already been mentioned as something they tried and it didn't work, forget about the advice you were going to offer.

A fundamental belief of the solution focused approach is the genuine recognition that each person is the 'expert' in their own life and is equipped with the knowledge to know what works for them. This is in contrast to other models where the worker is considered as the expert in 'fixing' the problems. The expertise of a solution focused worker is in structuring conversations to enable people to locate any knowledge, strengths, skills and abilities which will support them in achieving their hopes and wishes. This requires good communication skills, and discipline – resisting giving advice is difficult to do. We emphasise the importance of genuineness too, because workers can learn solution focused techniques but unless there is a sincere belief that those with whom you are working have the qualities and skills to achieve positive change, then workers may find themselves bringing knowledge and assumptions of understanding the 'problem' with them. Then they are in danger of imposing their own solutions and stifling people's cooperation and creativity.

PRACTICE ACTIVITY

Arthur had a cerebral embolism when he was 37. He has a supportive family and, after medical treatment, wanted to get his life going again. Before his embolism, Arthur had been hoping to build a deck behind his house, a task that now seemed impossible given his difficulty producing words, a considerable hand and arm tremor, and a marked degree of loss of motor power. Arthur still wished to do this despite the reservations of his surgeon and wife.

- As head of his rehabilitation team, what steps are necessary to enable Arthur to fulfil his goal?

- What outcomes would you expect for Arthur?

(Adapted from Brown and Brown 2003; see pp.154–158)

A further fundamental aspect of the solution focused approach is the appreciation that each person has the ability to identify the situation that they will be in when a problem has stopped happening, or is happening less often enough for it not to be so much of a problem. When the person has constructed what this will look like, this provides clear, concrete, person-centred, focused goals. Furthermore, these descriptions are best when they are solution-oriented, such as, 'I will be taking my medication on time,' in contrast to descriptions which are an absence of problems, such as, 'I will stop forgetting to take my medication.' Goal setting can also be undertaken on a group basis. Where there are problems with behaviour in group settings, it is possible to increase levels of respect and safer behaviour through exploring what a problem-free future looks like. To generate a description of what groups hope for and to establish clear, person-oriented goals, they can be asked questions such as:

- What makes a safe group?

- What does it look like?

- How is everyone behaving in this safe group?

- How are you talking to each other when you are in your safe group?

Individual and group strengths are identified so that people can be supported in maintaining a safe group, and they are asked to consider, 'How could you help someone when they need help to remember what is okay and not okay in your safer group?' Once these goals are defined, it is possible to locate exceptions, those times when the problems have not happened or happened less, focusing in great detail on where, when, who was involved and how it happened. For example, if people say that a safe group would be one where there isn't any bullying, the following questions could be asked:

- When there's no bullying, how will you be behaving instead?
- Can you tell me if any of this is happening already?
- Where does it happen?
- When does it happen?
- Who was doing this?
- How did it happen?
- Can you do more of this?

This sort of conversation can be very powerful and uplifting as it provides people with evidence that they have the resources, strengths and abilities to make the necessary changes in their lives. When people struggle to find times when they have overcome a difficulty that is troubling them or people who care for them, you can take a position of curiosity to consider times when the problems have happened less, and then ask scaled questions to build upon this.

CASE EXAMPLE

The idea that change is inevitable and happening all the time is helpful when talking with people who appear to have reached a plateau in their care management. They need every help and support to recognise small changes.

Shirley has had a period of intense rehabilitation following a severe subarachnoid haemorrhage. She feels that her progress has plateaued, and her loss of confidence and motivation has resulted in her not letting her husband out of her sight. When asked about tiny changes, he is able to help Shirley identify the times when she is already feeling confident and independent. She is able to brush her teeth, which is a small miracle considering her disabilities. Following on from recognising this achievement, Shirley is able to identify other tasks she is

> managing independently, all of which makes her feel more
> confident. (Adapted from Burns 2016, p.120)

As we mentioned earlier, solution focused practice was developed from asking people what worked for them (and discarding what they said doesn't work), therefore it is evidence-based. Its applicability in a wide range of situations and with people of all abilities has been demonstrated in a number of research studies, confirming the evidence base (for an overview, see Macdonald 2011). We turn now to demonstrate how the philosophy and practice of solution focused approaches link with the philosophy of the Workforce Strategy (DCSF 2008) and people's views on the sort of work and worker they find most helpful.

From solution focused philosophy to practice

Solution focused practice is aspirational in that it seeks to help and support people make better choices and lead rewarding lives in which they reach their full potential. In meeting with a person, the worker identifies the person's best hopes and goals. Where someone is not able to articulate these, the principles of the Care Act 2014 can provide appropriate goals (we explain how to help people with no speech or mental capacity to develop goals in detail in Chapter 2). Solution focused practice emphasises the importance of language and advocates a focus on the resources and skills and how these can contribute and assist the person in achieving their goal. People are expected to formulate realistic, achievable goals that are not harmful to themselves or others.

Participation – involving people in change

A solution focused approach supports people in the development of their own solutions to problems and difficulties through identifying and exploring those times when the problem or difficulty could have happened but didn't, or the person experienced the problem less. For example, when Steve worked with people who had committed sexual offences, his conversations were about the times when they could have sexually offended but didn't, searching for exactly what was different on these occasions so that they could learn from these successes in being non-offending. Looking for exceptions is important at any level of behaviour that is unacceptable, and we need to agree on what acceptable behaviour looks like for some people who may not be entirely clear about this.

PRACTICE ACTIVITIES

1. Next time you have to speak to someone about their behaviour, briefly express your concern about the behaviour and then ask:

   • Can you tell me if there have been any times when the behaviour didn't happen? (For example, can you tell me when you could have had a drink but chose not to?)

   • When did this happen?

   • Where did it happen?

   • How did you do it?

   • Was it hard or easy?

   • Do you think you can do it again?

   • Will you need any help to do it?

   • What sort of help will you need?

2. Next time you are trying to help someone who keeps getting a task wrong, briefly express your concern and then ask:

   • Have there been any times when you achieved the task? (For example, can you tell me if you ever managed to take your medication on time?) Or,

   • Can you tell me about any times when you almost managed the task? Or,

   • Can you tell me about any times when you succeeded in something that was hard when you first had a go?

   (Then go on to the questions in part 1.)

We are not interested in why problems occur or the nature of problems because we are too busy enabling people to find their solutions to difficulties. Neither is it necessarily useful to know why. Wittgenstein (1963, 1980) questioned the belief that there was a need to know the root of the problem in order to answer it. This may seem counterintuitive, but in our experience we have often found that people with whom we are working understand why they behave in a certain way and want support in finding ways to manage their behaviour/problem/difficulty differently. We have also found that people may not wish to, or feel unable to, explore the reasons why they are struggling, but do wish to change things. Digging into the problem, even with the best intentions, would clearly be disrespectful to that person, and possibly painful. However, the notion that 'you need to deal with the past before you can move on' is a powerful cultural and pop-psychological message, despite early psychoanalytic thinking questioning the usefulness of catharsis (Rycroft *et al.* 1966). In some instances, the notion can be dangerous.

CASE EXAMPLE

DM, a 40-year-old, single, pre-verbally profoundly deaf man, was receiving community support following psychiatric inpatient treatment some time previously. His social worker, newly qualified in working with deaf people, found D well and recommended that the psychiatrist stop his medication because he thought D's past problems related to his deafness as he had seldom had the chance to work through his feelings of frustration. The social worker sought advice on how to support the expression of frustration.

Although D was without speech, he had reasonable nonverbal language and was able to communicate by sign language and fingerspelling. The psychiatrist found it difficult to follow his train of thought as he was hallucinating and had numerous delusions and bizarre ideas, such as women leaving the screen when he was watching television and annoying him, and his left side telling him to do one thing while his right side told him another.

D was admitted to hospital and his medication resumed. His symptoms quickly disappeared. (Denmark 1994, pp.123–124)

We do find that some people expect to talk about the past with us and are puzzled when we focus on the future. Handling this expectation in a respectful way is important, and we find the most appropriate method of doing this with that person. For example, we might talk about increasing someone's immune system to inoculate them against future problems if this analogy works for them. You will notice throughout the examples in this book that we never ask a person 'why?' Should someone ask, 'Why?', we would ask what is more important to them: to have a solution or know why? For example, Bill was adamant that his problem could only be solved by discovering its cause, insisting that 'why' was more important to him than a solution. He was then asked: 'What will you be doing differently after we have discovered why you are like this?' He took a long time to answer, eventually straightening up and saying, 'I get it. There's no point digging in the graveyard when there are fresh fields to be ploughed.'

Furthermore, as de Shazer (1991) explicitly states, the solution is not necessarily related to the problem. Again this seems to run counter to common sense, but we find that when we listen very carefully to people and ask them what they think might work, they come up with solutions that have nothing to do with the problem. Neither are they solutions that we would ever have thought of, as the following solution shows.

CASE EXAMPLE

W. is a highly-intelligent 35-year-old man with autism. During his years as a student, he tried very hard to live up to the expectations of his surroundings, i.e. his friends, family, teachers. To do so, he often pushed his own limits and felt depressed as a result.

Once he graduated, he started looking for a job. In doing so, it was particularly difficult for him to keep an overview, to communicate and to interact with other people. W. has sensory processing issues, and he constantly feels overwhelmed by light and sound (he always experiences sound as 'noise').

After various unsuccessful work attempts, he decided that he did not find enough quality of life in living independently. He found it more useful to spend his time in another way and went to live with his mother again. His mother provided him with his daily needs: food, drinks and good advice.

As time went by, he started to exchange day and night: nowadays he is almost entirely nocturnal. He likes the dark and especially the quietness of the night. It enables him to concentrate on what he likes to do: he programmes video games, reads books and listens to his favourite music. Nobody drops in unexpectedly, everybody else in the house is asleep. His mother accepts his way of life, she notices he is happier that way. (Mattelin and Volckaert 2017)

CASE EXAMPLE

I remember just boarding a bus and I sat down and started singing quietly to myself a record that was currently in the charts. One of my voices said 'Oh no, not that old thing again.' And another voice chimed in too 'Yeah, I agree, why don't you sing something else?' So I asked them under my breath, 'Well, what do you want to hear?' And they said, 'Something from Elvis.' In response, I started singing 'We can't go on together with suspicious minds' and they sang along with me. In hindsight, I think that was pretty funny. (Williams 2003, p.6)

Participation – involving people in multi-agency work

People experience a sense of empowerment in response to our curiosity and style of conversation. A fundamental principle of solution focused ways of working is the notion of the worker not being responsible for, or the expert in, locating the problem or solution. Instead, their responsibilities and expertise lie in constructing a conversation which enables people to find their own solutions. This is more than just following a specific style of questioning. Each worker needs to believe genuinely that people do know best and are the experts in their own lives. We have found that this approach has been equally effective whether people are meeting with us voluntarily or under some form of coercion such as court orders.

The focus of work is away from working with deficits to working with capacity and capability. Nelson-Becker, Chapman and Fast (2013) talk about how older people have developed supportive networks and have a history of facing and succeeding with life's challenges, which are strengths they can call upon to meet the many inevitable losses associated with ageing.

We have found that effective multi-disciplinary working is underpinned by clarity and transparency by all participants so that people know what the professional concerns might be, thus providing them with the opportunity to respond constructively.

Transparency

Communication, and specifically how this is undertaken and its relevance and importance, is a key element of effective practice.

This fits with a central tenet of solution focused practice: the acknowledgement that language is of central importance, because how we talk about something generates a particular understanding of it. We have frequently experienced this in formal meetings where the language that is shared between professionals can be both judgemental and pathologising to people. This has a detrimental effect on people's motivation and affects their relationships with those professionals adversely. This is not to be misinterpreted as assuming that when someone has committed a crime or where someone has been hurt that this should not be challenged or addressed; quite the contrary. To increase motivation, change and safety, however, there needs to be a balance between identifying concerns alongside occasions when things have been different and better. It is possible to work within safeguarding frameworks and engage in transparent and respectful conversations.

White and Bateman (2008) suggest that it is: 'Helpful to see engagement as located in various actions which increase in the relationship between people as they get to know each other and learn to value what they have to offer to each other' (p.18). Such 'actions' would include honest and transparent practice, giving people time and opportunities and (as practitioners) reflecting on what we could do differently to support and achieve increased levels of engagement. Finding a way to communicate with people is essential in helping them locate a voice, and ultimately their full participation. This is a very obvious statement, but from discussions with both practitioners and people, locating a language can be difficult.

CASE EXAMPLE

Susan was at risk of her children being taken in care as a result of her neglect of them. As part of the proceedings, she was subject to a psychological assessment, which concluded that she had a mental age of eight and therefore was not fit to plead in court. Overwhelmed by the occasion and formality of the questions, Susan had not been able to express herself at all well so the story of her unhappy circumstances went unheard. These circumstances included: being subject to domestic abuse by her boyfriend (who did not live with her), being alienated from her family at the instigation of her boyfriend, and being verbally and physically abused by neighbours. Not surprisingly, she was deeply depressed.

Enlisting the support of her family and moving her to a house nearer to them resulted in a rapid improvement in Susan's mood – and cognitive ability. She became able to talk about her hopes for herself and her children, and what help she would need to achieve these. A later assessment estimated that she was functioning at the level of a 14-year-old.

Assessment

It is also important to acknowledge people's wishes that their strengths be recognised. We find that a consistent emphasis on strengths increases people's motivation to work with us, so, on initial contact, we will ask questions about what is going right and what people are good at. This can be a surprise to many people who are often expecting to be viewed as full of problems, and, indeed, might view themselves as such. In solution focused practice, talk of strengths is important because despite life's struggles, everyone possesses strengths that can be used to improve the quality of their lives. Workers should respect these strengths and the directions in which people wish to apply them: 'When we consider the stresses under which many service users live, we have to be impressed with their ability to keep going, perhaps not all the time, but more often than we give them credit' (Howe 2008, p.101).

PRACTICE ACTIVITY

Konika has a very miserable home life where she is constantly denigrated but she needs to be financially dependent on her family for another year. Her misery takes the form of a feeling that she is possessed by the voices of her family, which are preventing her from building on the few exceptions she is able to identify. For example she says:

> I didn't feel like crying, just six days…just nothing to cry about. I don't feel six days not crying is much strength. More like six months. It's self-pity, that's all it is. Little things coming into my head and bring me sadness… Like I drop down a hole. All these things come from nowhere and push me in.

- What questions could you ask that might inspire Konika to climb out of her hole?

Focusing on strengths turns workers away from the temptation to judge or blame people for their difficulties and towards discovering how they have managed to survive, even in the most difficult of circumstances. All environments – even the most bleak – contain resources, maintains Saleebey (2013). We find that talking about strengths frequently decreases levels of anxiety in people, particularly in situations where people have behaved badly and are preparing for an onslaught of negativity from professionals and carers. Instead, they hear things that people think they are good at. As a solution focused assumption is that problems are never always there – change is constant – and that people will always have some strengths, we can genuinely ask questions that will find real exceptions.

We are also aware through conversations with people at the end of our work that engagement has increased due to their experiencing a feeling of empowerment to remain as the experts in their own lives. For example, parents can experience too much negativity when their children are behaving badly and pass this on to the child by becoming angry and disappointed in them. Judith bypasses this by ending her initial strengths conversation with the comment: 'I don't know what you have been doing with [name of child] but with all these good points you must have been doing something seriously right.' This frees the parents up to join with the child against the problem, using all the strengths, resources, qualities, skills and so on that you have discovered. Recognising parents' competences is also important where they are looking after a sick child.

CASE EXAMPLE

The nurses have been brilliant...his nasogastric tube came out again, a week later. But he was brilliant. He let me put it in! ... Amy and Sarla let me try and reassured me it wouldn't hurt Sam. They said if he got stressed or if I didn't like it, I could stop and they'd give me a hand. And he sat there and Amy said: 'Go on, swallow!' And Sam did, you know. And it went straight down. They talked about things with me and Sam and it was so fine.

And Amy brought me all the things to show me about his gastrostomy and about having a Mickey button put in. And she said they could put the Mickey button in and measure him up... and they could show me...but I just didn't feel that I could take that on – not at the moment anyway. So they said, 'no worries, no hurry' – so I can get that in a week or something – once I thought about it – got my head round it and things... It's all a lot to take on you know.

But yeah, they've been really good. Just there in the end of the phone. If you just want to talk and that. And they don't tell me what to do – not unless I really ask them that – they find out what I want and then we sort it out. Nothing's a trouble. They don't make me frightened – nothing like that – just calm and not winding the situation up. Sam's hard enough work as it is without everyone telling me 'do this do that'... You can ask them anything, anything at all. They talk things through and I can tell them if I don't think something will work right with Sam. They are really experienced but Sam's a really special child – he needs things done a special way and I know what he needs. (Carter 2007, p.68)

PRACTICE ACTIVITY

- Explore one of the things that is most meaningful in your life by asking yourself, a family member and a friend (separately): What is the thing that is the most meaningful to me in my life?

- Compare the three responses and ask yourself, which rings the most true?

- How could you use these questions with carers and cared for people?

(Brown and Brown 2003, p.85)

Feedback

Constructive feedback is vital at whatever level of contact with a person, be this a certificate of achievement from an employer, copies of therapeutic notes, or the minutes of a review meeting. This is not simply praise, it is about identifying people's competence and sense of being in control of their lives and able to solve their problems. Any sport instructor will tell you that people learn most quickly when they practise their successes and become disheartened when they have to repeat their failed attempts. This is because practising their successes increases their motivation, uses their skills, and helps them to work out what they are doing right so that they can do more of it.

Safeguarding

A solution focused approach can also be adopted within an adult protection framework and the responsibilities, both to the person with whom you are working and the wider community, which come with this. Turnell and Edwards (1999) devised a Signs of Safety approach in child protection as a comprehensive (risk) assessment which documents both concerns and safety alongside canvassing the goals and perspectives of both professionals and family members. In child protection work, the main solution focus is on developing and increasing the level of safety, thus parents and children are required to demonstrate behaviour which is measurably safe.

We think that this approach has merits with other situations broader than just child protection. The way that the assessment is structured enables parents to understand others' concerns alongside an acknowledgement of strengths and positive attributes. This facilitates transparency and an understanding of what needs to be different for professionals to no longer be concerned.

One technique is to use the Three Houses model (www.mythreehouses.com), where people are invited to state what is going well; what they are worried about; and what they ideally want in a problem-free future (hopes and dreams). Everyone's concerns are listed and everyone has a clear idea of what will be different when there is sufficient safety. Strengths are identified as resources to create more safety for vulnerable people. The worker will then begin to document things that they have already heard as well as asking questions such as, 'Since this came to light, what have you done differently to increase safety?' The information that is shared (in response to these questions) is noted down in another column headed 'Safety'.

As these questions are asked and there is a recognition from families that we are not going to blame, or *tell* them what they need to be doing, but rather are intent on building on the levels of safety that are already visible, there is a noticeable difference in their motivation to engage with the worker and the process, alongside a reduction in feelings of anxiety.

It is clear from the outset that if we have any concerns about the welfare of their own or other children that this information will be shared with the local authority. For example, where there are few, or no, signs of safety, concern is obviously increased and external safeguarding measures need to be instituted.

CASE EXAMPLE

Viktor is a 57-year-old cabinet maker who has been married to Valerie for 35 years. A fortnight ago, he accosted his local priest in the street, accusing him of having an affair with Valerie. Two days ago, he burst into Valerie's workplace, hitting her boss around the head and then walking out. Valerie's boss didn't want to make a formal complaint but asked her not to come into work until 'something is done' about Viktor. Valerie is the epitome of a downtrodden woman.

Viktor's best hopes are for Valerie to admit her affairs and stop them, and for the plot which is preventing his cabinet designs from being recognised to be stopped. He knows that Valerie is having affairs because her leg movements in sleep mean that she is having an orgasm. He is not sure where the plot to deny him recognition as a cabinet maker comes from, so he has brought a box full of his drawings, which he spreads out to make his point. Whenever he is asked a question, he returns to these two preoccupations, so he is asked: 'If 0 is you have some doubt that your ideas are correct and 100 is you know for certain that they are, where are you on this scale?' Viktor placed himself at 100. (Although there could be some very slight consolation that he had actually answered a question for the first time, this is not sufficient to overrule the issue of Valerie's safety.)

Viktor was referred to the community mental health team, which decided that he did not warrant compulsory admission to hospital, and he not surprisingly refused voluntary treatment – the suspicion and mistrust that go hand in hand with paranoia made it very unlikely. Valerie's adult daughters were contacted and they convinced her that she needed to leave Viktor for her own safety. When seen some weeks later, she looked a completely different, brighter person. The outcome for Viktor was less happy.

PRACTICE ACTIVITIES

1. Think of someone with whom you are working or have worked where there are safeguarding concerns:

    *   What could you write in the three houses of 'Going Well'; 'Concerns'; and 'Hopes and Dreams'?

    *   How might this help in formulating a safety plan to reduce risk?

    *   What would your safety plan look like?

2. Following a stroke, Lena's husband became her carer. After his death, Lena became dependent on her teenage son, Mark, for most of her physical care. She has had several hospital admissions following overdoses and falls. Her current admission raises safety concerns as she has a black eye. She complained to neighbours previously that her son hit her but denies this in hospital. She both loves and fears her son but is confused about how she wants to live her life. She doesn't want to put Mark out as he still owes rent arrears on his previous flat and would have to sofa surf.

- Draw up a preliminary safety plan which will meet the needs of both Lena and Mark.

Summary

- Solution focused practice is especially appropriate for the adult workforce because it is strengths-based, participatory and transparent and, above all, it is fundamentally ambitious for every person.

- The philosophy underpinning solution focused practice includes an unwavering belief in people's capacities to find their own solutions. The guiding principle is: if it works, do more of it; if it doesn't work, do something different.

- The techniques provide a discipline within which the worker can remain true to the philosophy and principle. Macdonald (2011) found solution focused practice to work equally well with problems such as anorexia, autism, violence, pain, substance misuse and mental illnesses, regardless of learning ability, and with long-lasting results.

Key points

- Don't trust your own theories about anyone; remain *curious* about how people are different.

- Do believe that people already know what they can do and are able to do it – it's just that sometimes they don't realise this. Help them to see it by asking helpful questions.

- The problem is the problem; get the people working against *it* with you.

- It's not a problem if it has no solution (at least, it is not a problem to be changed, only to be coped with).

- We don't need to understand the problem in order to understand the solution, unless it is a purely physical matter or a question of medication.

- Don't worry about people resisting change – encourage them to resist the problem.

- Use lots of scaled questions, with 10 = perfect and 0 = the pits.

- Don't take too much responsibility. Responsibility is like a cake: the more you eat, the less there is for the other person. Your responsibility mainly includes asking questions that invite them to take more of the cake.

- There is always something about everyone that is okay; spend some time thinking about what that is, because it can fix what is not okay. No problem is ever 100 per cent bad always, so talk about *exceptions* to problems.

- Rather than looking for more understanding of the problem, look instead at what people are *doing well*.

- Slow down – go back to what the person hopes for (has any of that ever happened before? What coping strategies worked in the past?). The more time you spend on their strengths and successes the better. Compliment them on coping *in spite of* all they have to endure.

- Remember that a solution may well not be related to a problem.

- Avoid negativity by only asking a question to which you do *not* know the answer, i.e. don't ask, 'How are you?' if you know the answer will be, 'Awful.' Instead, ask, 'What's better since we last met?' If the answer is, 'Nothing,' ask, 'What was better just after we met?' 'What was better the next day?' 'What was better this morning?' This conveys that you are more interested in what is better than in what is worse or the same.

- We can make a possibility more possible by talking, imagining and figuring out how to start it. This means talking in detail about what it will be like, what the person will be doing, how the person will feel, what other people will notice, etc. (see Milner, Myers and O'Byrne 2015).

We address each one of these key points in more detail in the subsequent chapters.

Chapter Two

Taking People Seriously

This chapter looks at the first, and possibly the most important, skill needed in working with adults: effective communication and engagement. In other words, getting off to a good start. Underpinning all solution focused practice is the basic principle of treating people as worth doing business with, respecting them in their own right – even when you don't like them. This is not as self-evident as it sounds. Professionals talk about the importance of being person-centred; of engaging with people to build up a relationship; being culturally sensitive; and, of being respectful. Being person-centred, however, can be a suspiciously catch-all phrase which does little to help the busy health or care worker communicate with people effectively.

CASE EXAMPLE

I felt fairly confident in talking to people but what I realized when I was doing the course (in solution focused practice) and afterwards, was that I had no direction. There was a lot of waffling going on, I let people waffle a hell of a lot. I was a good listener, yes, I could listen for England. This could go on for weeks with no solution in sight. (Nurse C. in Bowles, Mackintosh and Torn 2001, p.352)

Effective communication

How best to communicate has been largely influenced by person-centred and psycho-social counselling literature. The person-centred approach has its origins in the work of Carl Rogers, who set out the conditions of a therapeutic relationship: being non-directive, congruent, and having unconditional regard for people and empathy.

Rogers stressed that being person-centred is a process in which the core conditions overlap, not a set of instructions, and the process is not meant to lead to goals.

Over the years, distortions of what he actually said have crept in as person-centred counsellors integrated other methods into their work, with the core conditions incorporated into communication skills taught as separate qualities. For example, 'empathy' is a common component of communication training involving teaching the worker to be able to sense the person's world as if it were their own, and this is seen as an important (and often uncritical) component of communication. More contemporary approaches include the concept of emotional intelligence (Goleman 1995), which claims to have identified the key qualities required to work effectively with people through:

> the capacity to reason about emotions, and of emotions to enhance thinking. It includes the abilities to accurately perceive emotions, to access and generate emotions so as to assist thought, to understand emotions and emotional knowledge, and to reflectively regulate emotions so as to promote emotional and intellectual growth. (Mayer et al. 2004, p.197)

It will be obvious that this raises many questions about how this is done, as emotions are notoriously difficult to judge and make sense of. Emotional intelligence remains a contested concept that can be rather woolly and also depends on the presumption that people's emotions are relatively straightforward to observe, understand and categorise, whereas we consider this to be an extremely difficult task that is prone to the projection of your own interpretation onto the behaviour of others.

The psycho-social approach has its origins in the psychoanalytic work of Sigmund and Anna Freud as a means to understand seemingly irrational behaviour and gain insight. This approach, too, has been (over)simplified and developed into psycho-social counselling as opposed to psychoanalysis. In psycho-social counselling, it is axiomatic that people are only truly engaged through the development of a therapeutic relationship and that this relationship will:

- take time to develop
- probably be resisted

- include the person saying things that are not necessarily what they mean

- involve gentle interpretative challenges.

(For an overview of person-centred and psycho-social approaches, see Milner and O'Byrne 2004.)

One problem with this is that the worker becomes the expert on what is going on in other people's minds. And it is only too easy to get it completely wrong. We naturally look at things from our own perspective and filter what they tell us through our favourite theories and knowledge. These are likely to be concerned with long-term dangers to health and welfare, such as smoking, substance misuse and obesity. People, of course, look at things from their own perspective and are much more likely to be concerned about how their diminished physical and mental health abilities affect everyday relationships, the humiliation arising from loss of independence, and often hopelessness. Their carers also look at things from their own perspective, which may differ from both the person they care for and the worker.

CASE EXAMPLE

Maureen's younger brother Ross has Down's syndrome. Maureen had always been very close to him and had promised their mother that, when she died, Maureen would continue to care for him. After their mother's death Ross moved in with his sister.

At the age of 49 Ross developed Alzheimer's-type dementia. Maureen continued to look after him but her own health began to fail as Ross became more disabled and demanding of her time. Maureen refused all offers of help. She wanted to honour the promise she had given to her mother and she worried that no one else would love and care for her brother as she did. Only when the situation was at breaking point was Ross given a place in a small residential house. His sister felt that she had been a complete failure.

Maureen was left in emotional turmoil with mixed and confusing feelings towards the staff. On the one hand she felt enormous gratitude to staff at the home; on the other hand she had a constant nagging doubt about their care and worried that they did not give Ross sufficient care and love. Her worries and anxieties were exacerbated by the changes she saw in Ross. His deteriorating condition made her anxious that this may be because of the lack of staff time and attention rather than the inevitable consequence of the condition. (Kerr 2007, p.163)

Marriott (2003) explores the mixed feelings that carers often have about their situation, including those that they may find difficult to admit to others, such as thoughts of murder. He also talks frankly, and often amusingly, about subjects that are difficult to talk about with health and social care workers, such as sex, (in)continence, hurtful comments and changed relationships in which the carer is

> *not just as important as they are [the cared for person]. Why are we expected to sacrifice ourselves for someone else? And, yes, I mean sacrifice. We're not talking about giving up five minutes of time once or twice a week. Another holiday from this year to the next. We're talking about changing our entire way of life. The old wasn't perfect, but it was the best we could do. The new one isn't even ours. It is someone else's life. And it's one that doesn't suit at all. (p.34)*

Bowles *et al.* (2001) remark that despite non-directive counselling techniques forming the backbone of communication skills programmes, they have little utility at the bedside where lack of time and the emotional cost of entering the patient's private world means that nurses often protect themselves by blocking communication through abrupt changes of subject or focusing on the least threatening aspect of a conversation (for an overview of the research, see Bowles *et al.* 2001). It is probable that care home workers similarly protect themselves as, like nurses, they often experience high task demands, low levels of job control and inadequate support.

PRACTICE ACTIVITY

- On a scale of 0–10, how confident are you in talking with people who are troubled?

- On a scale of 0–10, how competent are you in talking with people who are troubled?

- On a scale of 0–10, how willing are you to talk with people who are troubled?

Take your lowest score and ask yourself what you will be doing differently when that score goes up one point.

Central to the essential components of person-centred counselling is the idea that the therapeutic relationship is where change happens. The danger here is that the person's real world of relationships with family and friends is marginalised. This is an enormous waste of vital resources as well as adding a tremendous burden on the worker to fix everything. As we saw in the previous chapter, solution focused practice is very different:

- It does not assume that engaging people is difficult.

- It does not try to replace important people in people's lives. Instead, it recruits them as important members of the person's helping team.

- It does not worry about 'resistance'. In solution focused practice, resistance is considered to be just that: a protest that tells us that we haven't yet found out how the person wishes to be supported, so we need to discover their unique way of cooperating.

- It does not assume that the relationship will necessarily be lengthy; instead, it views the relationship as short term, collaborative and transitional until its purpose is fulfilled.

- The relationship must be transparent and genuinely two-way.

- It can be applied to work in any setting; for example, Unwin 2005 (GP practice); Macdonald 2011 (psychiatry); Milner and Myers 2016 (violence and confrontation); Jacob 2001 (eating disorders); Burns 2016 (speech therapy); Ghul 2015 (occupational therapy); and nursing: 'solution focused practice is culturally congruent with nursing practice as it focuses on wellness and health, not pathology, and is oriented to towards empowering the patient to recognize their own strengths and competence' (Bowles *et al.* 2001).

Respecting people

Health and social care workers don't need sophisticated counselling skills to show respect for people who simply want us to listen carefully, without trivialising; to be available and accessible, with regular and predictable contact; to be accepting, explaining and suggesting options and choices; to be realistic, reliable and straight talking; and to be trustworthy in terms of confidentiality and consulting with them before taking action. Beresford (2007) found that older people valued advice and advocacy, negotiation with agencies and services, signposting and other practical guidance as well as psycho-therapeutic support. It is clear from this that it doesn't matter how accurate your empathy is if you fail to be punctual, reliable, courteous and trustworthy.

Many people with mania or other psychosis have an extensive knowledge of medications and can recollect which ones they found most useful. Often their chosen medication will be effective once again. If not, they are more open to try professional suggestions if their own opinions have been respected first. They may need some calming medication in the first place but even when still disturbed, respectfulness is not only possible but helps you obtain a good outcome as this case example from Alasdair Macdonald shows.

CASE EXAMPLE

This patient of mine was a housewife in her mid-30s, childless, with a history of one previous episode of mania in another part of the UK. She was admitted from home to our Psychiatric Intensive Care ward under certificate after some days of gross overactivity and disinhibited behaviour (e.g. walking out into the traffic). She and others reported reduced appetite, reduced sleep and impaired concentration. She had always been vivacious and energetic (e.g. cleaning her whole house every week).

On admission she was only able to keep to question and answer for three to four minutes at a time. She did not regard herself as ill. In response to the solution focused scaling questions: 'Where are you on a scale of 0–10?' 'I'm at 20!' 'What number would your husband say?' 'Oh, he would say 7.' 'And your GP?' 'He might say 5.' She agreed that these others might sometimes be more accurate than she, so she agreed to work towards these people saying 'maybe 9 and see how it goes'.

The ward staff encouraged her to use some of her energy and housework skills in assisting the ward cleaner. We held a weekly ward meeting of all staff, in which the patient would be invited in to give her views after the staff discussion. During this meeting, she burst in uninvited and sprayed all the staff with furniture polish. Luckily her excitement reduced her ability to aim, and most of the polish went onto the back or the top of heads, with less risk of injury to staff. She was then ushered out of the room, using Home Office approved Control and Restraint procedures, to be invited back ten minutes later to discuss our proposed treatment plan. She was able to tell us which medication had been most helpful, in her opinion, during the previous episode. She responded well to calming medication and was soon able to move to an open ward prior to discharge. (Alasdair Macdonald, personal communication)

Explaining yourself

If conversations are to be useful, people need to know the purpose of them. They need to know what we can and cannot do, when and where we will do it, what our and other people's concerns are, details of any rules and boundaries, how long it is likely to take, and where we can be contacted.

Then we would check that the information we had been given on the person was accurate. We have found these conversations helpful as they encourage transparency and put the work in a context. Furthermore, we hope that on a longer-term basis this will provide another way that people and their families can think and respond to difficulties outside our work with them, as well as shifting their own family conversations to considering each other's strengths as an alternative to recognising each other's weaknesses. As Unwin (2005) comments, it's better to have a GP waiting room full of heroes instead of being full of problems.

CASE EXAMPLE

Nurse: Hello Sam, remember me, I'm Jane. Thanks for talking yesterday about the surgery that is planned. We talked a lot. You showed that you have a good understanding of the actual procedure as well as the risks associated with it. We also talked about the anxious feelings you have. As we agreed yesterday, today we will be spending some time getting to know your situation more deeply, what your concerns are, as well as your goals in working together with me. How does that sound?

Sam: That sounds okay. What would you like to know?

Jane: Well, there's a lot I don't know, and I'm not an expert on you, you are. But I guess a good place to begin would be with our situation, our relationship right now. Sam, I wonder if you could tell me, what needs to come out of this meeting so that you can say this is helpful?

Sam: I don't know. Maybe to feel less anxious, to feel like I can take charge of these jangly nerves, I don't know, to feel more confident that I think I can get through this.

Jane: Okay, so it sounds like what you want is to feel more in control of the Jangly Nerves. Let's look at these Jangly Nerves in closer detail.

(McAllister 2007, p.41)

Where you are having solution focused conversations makes some difference, but not a lot. You don't necessarily need a special room. Many of you will find that you are talking with people in busy wards, chaotic homes, clinics, or even while taking a walk with a person. A group of well-child nurses even held solution focused telephone conversations with families unable to attend their clinic (Polaschek and Polaschek 2007).

You don't necessarily need to take people off to a quiet room; it is perfectly possible to have a useful conversation in any environment, although when you are dealing with a group of people, it is helpful to build in occasional individual sessions. For example, a solution focused group pain management programme also included a monthly drop-in session with an occupational therapist (Simm, Iddon and Barker 2014).

Alternatively, you could let people know how to signal when they want to talk with you one-to-one. For parents who may well be busy preparing a meal or emptying the washing machine when a child wishes to talk with them, we suggest a secret sign, such as moving an ornament slightly (Milner and Bateman 2011) but agreeing a signal for adults is more problematic. For example, hospital patients have only a buzzer to press when they want help or to talk about their concerns. This is a crude method of communication and the busy nurse may well not be pleased to be signalled for something less than an urgent physical need.

PRACTICE ACTIVITY

- Other than pressing the buzzer, how can patients be enabled to signal that they want to talk but that it could wait until the nurse is less busy?

- How can domiciliary workers make it simple for people to contact them?

CASE EXAMPLE

Tremayne is in danger of losing his tenancy in supported housing due to complaints from neighbours. He often has friends round in the evening and they are very rowdy. When asked to keep the noise down, Tremayne becomes verbally abusive. Letting friends stay over also breaches his tenancy agreement. Having partied late, Tremayne then sleeps most of the day and doesn't answer the door.

He has not replied to a letter from his housing support worker asking him to make an appointment to talk about things. From discussion with the annoyed neighbours, the worker found out that after his friends arrive, Tremayne usually goes to a local off-licence, so his worker waylaid him on his next trip to the off-licence and held a solution focused conversation with him as they walked along. It transpired that Tremayne didn't actually want friends over but he found it difficult to say no when they arrived. The worker offered Tremayne a letter to show to his friends, outlining the tenancy agreement, but Tremayne didn't think this would deter them. He decided simply not to answer the door.

Problem-free talk

If, as solution focused practitioners, we believe that people have the ability to find their own solutions to problems, then we must also be clear about how we will set about finding out how they will 'do' their solutions. Unlike problem-solving approaches where the professional already has the answer, it is quite possible that a person doesn't yet know that they have a solution. After all, vulnerable adults are more likely to be given information than consulted, and to be asked for advice even more rarely.

Solution focused practice is ambitious for people, so it is important to set each person up to succeed by engaging with them as people, not as problems. We ask about their hobbies, interests, hopes, aspirations, what they enjoy doing, what are they good at, what the hardest thing they have ever done is and so on. This is not idle chit-chat; we are genuinely curious to learn more about the person with whom we are talking. When they tell us things such as that they enjoy gardening or reading to grandchildren, we ask more curious questions, such as:

- When did you find out that you are good at reading aloud and keeping a child interested?

- How do you help your grandchild to choose what you will read?

- Do you research books suitable for your grandchildren?

- What's the best bit of reading aloud?

- How did you get to be so good at it?

What we are trying to do in these sorts of conversations is find out about the personal qualities of the person. This is not the same as looking for positives; it is about identifying and highlighting abilities, competences and skills. Once a person's competences are noticed, it is easier to get a solution going. The pain management programme mentioned earlier paid attention to competences: 'There is also a support group (Pain Clinic Plus) that meets twice weekly, led by *expert* patients...and a wellbeing choir run by a pain patient for pain patients (*her expertise* as a singing teacher has been noticed and utilised!)' (Simm *et al.* 2014, p.52, our emphasis).

CASE EXAMPLE

There is one woman in the [hearing voices] group, Julia, who talks about how she always thinks the neighbours are talking about her. In one of the meetings Julia mentioned that she'd done a lot of gardening on the previous weekend. I said to her, 'well it was a lovely day wasn't it – I bet there were a lot of people around'. And she replied, 'yes all the neighbours were out, some were having a barbecue'. When I asked Julia how long she was gardening for, she said 'about three hours', and so I asked her, 'in those three hours, did you think other people were talking about you?' And she said, 'Come to think of it now, I didn't.' We went on to explore why this was and we heard Julia describe how doing the gardening, focusing on the plants and on the small details, meant that she was free from paranoia during that time. (Bullimore 2003, p.26)

PRACTICE ACTIVITIES

1. The questions asked of the woman who enjoys reading to her grandchildren will reveal several skills and personal qualities which may well be transferable to other aspects of her life:

    •   Make a list of at least ten of them which may be possible in this scenario.

2. Next time you have a conversation with a person you know well, pretend that you have just met them and are curious to find out all about them. Ask lots of questions, such as:

    •   What is the hardest thing you have ever done?

    •   If your pet could talk, what would it tell me about you?

    •   If you could borrow someone's life for the day, whose would it be?

    •   What good thing do you do that no one has noticed?

    •   What was the best time you ever had?

Curious listening

When we ask trainees to list their skills, they almost always head their lists with 'I'm a good listener' but find it difficult to expand on this and say how they 'do listening' and how their listening is effective. Communications literature has much to say on how to listen and give feedback but not much on what we are supposed to be listening *to* when we hold conversations. This is because as professionals we tend to believe that we know better than the lay person so we often interrupt them, tell them what they are thinking, what they 'really' mean and what they should be doing: 'We have all been accused of failing to listen to our nearest and dearest. Those less nearly related may be too polite and fail to correct us when we need it most' (Ross 1996, p.92). We find it odd that workers who are in charge of the agenda for the conversation then talk about listening with a 'third ear' for what the person might be trying to convey by their body language.

Solution focused practice makes no effort to listen for what is *not* being said on the grounds that there may well be nothing to read between the lines. Instead, we listen carefully at the level of the word by:

- Noting idiosyncratic use of language, repeated words, language that sticks out.

- Inquiring about any word or phrase that appears to have special meaning for the person.

- Checking that we have the same meaning of the word and/or picture used; this is especially important when people have picked up formal language from professionals.

- Not changing the words people use in our conversations or reports, making sure that the conversation is developing from their own words, not our own.

- Only asking questions to which we do not think we know the answer.

- Listening to the reply to one question before deciding what our next question is going to be.

- Asking if we are asking questions that are interesting/relevant to them.

- Asking if there are any questions we haven't asked that are important to them.

This is not to say that we don't have an agenda; we do, but we are clear and transparent about what our hopes are for the work. In the case of adult safeguarding, we need to see what is happening for us to be confident that safety has increased, and that we don't need to work together any more so that we can recommend closing the case. We are listening for skills, competences, abilities, strengths and resiliences because these are the qualities that will be used in the solution. People like this type of conversation, making it much easier to engage their attention and cooperation. It is also less emotionally draining for the professional.

Bowles *et al.* (2001) introduced solution focused training to a group of nurses who agreed that, prior to this, they had 'not considered that there might be an alternative to problem-dominated talk, other than to avoid interpersonal engagement…one nurse said "I dreaded clinic, because it was so depressing…it was very much doom and gloom and depressing"' (p.351). After solution focused training, the same nurse commented: 'I think it's empowered me. It's released me from this awful feeling that as a nurse I have to put a plaster on and sort of send them away' (p.352).

There are also some things we deliberately don't do when we hold solution focused conversations. We don't:

- Interpret what they are saying or check what they are saying against a favourite theory.

- Ask 'why'; if people knew why they were doing something damaging to their health or welfare, they either wouldn't do it or would be embarrassed to admit that they did.

PRACTICE ACTIVITY

Jane is a young woman with mild learning difficulties who is experiencing problems with alcohol and drugs. She often looks neglected and unkempt and when this has been raised, Jane has become very angry and confrontational with her carers. She spent most of her childhood in care following physical abuse by her mother and father, and she has been diagnosed with dyslexia, dyspraxia and ADHD, which was treated with the powerful stimulant, Ritalin. As a black woman, Jane has received a great deal of racist abuse in the area where she lives and also in her past when she was placed with white foster carers for a time. Jane has recently started a relationship with a white woman, Sharon, who is significantly older than Jane and also has intermittent problems with alcohol:

- When reading this example, what range of explanations for the situation can you identify?

- Where have your explanations come from?

- How do your explanations help to inform intervention to assist Jane?

Using humour and playfulness

Problems have a knack of convincing adults that it's time to get down to the serious business of problem-solving. This approach also has the danger of making the person *the problem* rather than seeing them as someone *with a problem*. But, as C. Murray Parkes says (1986), death is too serious a matter to be taken solemnly; thus, there is room for humour in solution focused practice, however serious the situation. Being playful means using humour as a means of engaging people – sharing laughter is a much quicker way of connecting with a person than is establishing 'accurate empathy' as long as it 'is humour that builds people up, reduces hierarchy or makes the problem look small and ridiculous' (Sharry, Madden and Darmody 2001, p.34). The nurse mentioned earlier who dreaded clinic, later says of solution focused practice:

> *Now I have permission to laugh with patients in clinics. A lot of my patients have chronic problems that I cannot do anything about and to have permission to sort of, okay not trivialize it, but bring some humour into it, to balance it out with a positive, you know, 'What's your good day like?' It makes, yes, it's lightened the load. (Bowles et al. 2001, pp.352–353)*

Giving information

Workers often have an education role, seeing communication as a means of giving information. We all like to be helpful so when we are faced with a person with a problem we are tempted to share our expertise and advise them what to do, whether it is a mother having problems with breast feeding, a man who loses his temper and hits his partner, a young adult who misuses substances, an overweight person whose diabetes is not well controlled and so on. This is not an effective way of educating a person for a number of reasons:

- It ignores the person's own knowledge. Some people may want to be given information but many will already have a great deal of knowledge gleaned from personal experience, internet searches, and family and friends. This needs to be explored, not only to save you time in repeating information but also to check out the accuracy of it.

- It ignores the person's experience. The advice given may be irrelevant to the person's life situation. Men on domestic violence programmes frequently complained to us that the scenarios given won't work for them. For example, Jack was advised to walk away from aggression at bus stops. Not only did he never catch a bus – where he lived had very few buses and had a high level of violence – but he would be the target of violence should he be known not to stand up to it. Similarly, Virgil was advised to overtake lone women at night so as not to seem as though he was following them. He lived in an area of high drug crime and prostitution where it would be inappropriate to overtake lone women late at night.

- It neglects the reality that there is a gap between knowing what you ought to do and actually doing it. We remember talking with a group of health visitors who had just completed a course on nutrition and were keen to incorporate the knowledge into their practice. We asked how many of them had changed *their* eating habits as a result of the course – not one.

- It is not tailored to individual education needs. As any teacher will tell you, it's more effective to teach *the child* how to do maths, not teach *maths* to the child.

In solution focused practice, set programmes are not used. The worker's stance is that of an 'expert by invitation', sharing expertise with the person to build towards their preferred future *where invited*. Questions are used that search out individual, and group, education needs and existing expertise; for example:

- Is there anything you need to know about resolving/managing your situation?

- What things have you already tried that have worked?

- What things have you tried but weren't suitable for your situation?

And this approach works. Cui *et al.* (2008) conducted a randomised controlled study of 60 people with type 2 diabetes, where half received a combined education and solution focused practice programme and half received conventional health education. The group in the combined education and solution focused practice scored significantly higher in knowledge and skill of self-care, compliance with doctors and clinical satisfaction. Their blood sugar and blood pressure levels were also significantly reduced.

Similarly, in a 'living well despite pain' programme, the ethos is solution focused but participants share experiences of their pain and the impact this has on their lives. Facilitators allow space and time for listening and acknowledgement. Their curiosity and questions lie not in investigating the problem but rather in continuing to notice strengths and possibilities. In this sense, the group is solution focused but not problem phobic. Participants described that the future-oriented focus and commitment to follow-up helped them to feel reassured and that they didn't feel 'dumped':

> *Importantly, for many participants, being able to exercise this independence and self-determination in practice appeared to facilitate an enhanced sense of self-understanding, particularly with regard to which aspects of their chronic condition were within their control and a sense of acceptance about what elements of change were possible:*

> *I've started to accept that I've got it [chronic pain] not because I've done anything wrong or bad in my life...it's taught me to cope a lot better with it, it's taught me that it can't be cured but it's not the worst thing in the world [...] now I couldn't have said that three or four months back. (Dargan, Simm and Murray 2014, p.39)*

Working with people you don't like

It's all very well talking about respecting people and treating them as people worth doing business with but it can be incredibly difficult when you are faced with someone whose behaviour disgusts you, or where they are simply unnecessarily nasty to you, or where they don't seem to make any effort to help themselves, or they promise to stop a behaviour only to do it again repeatedly.

PRACTICE ACTIVITY

Choose one of the scenarios below and ask yourself what annoys you most about that situation:

1. Following a stroke, Norman has been admitted to a care home on the estate where he has lived all his life.

Although he can walk with a Zimmer frame and feed himself, he is unable to wash himself. One of the carers recognises him as the caretaker at her junior school where he sexually abused her cousin. No action was taken as her cousin was not prepared to make a statement. The carer cannot bring herself to undertake Norman's physical care.

2. Helen's support worker is coming out of family court care proceedings to remove Helen and her partner, Danny's, children where the support worker has given evidence of the effect on Helen of Danny's domestic violence. As she passes Helen and Danny, who are arm in arm, Danny gives her a hard stare and makes a throat-cutting movement with his hand.

3. Weighing 160 kilos, Collette is hoping to be accepted for gastric band surgery. You have been asked to assess her suitability for this surgery. On asking her about what changes she intends making to her lifestyle in preparation for, and following surgery, she looks at you in amazement, saying she doesn't eat much anyway and she's never liked exercise.

4. Ayesha's arms are covered in scars from where she has repeatedly cut herself. She says that she doesn't want to cut herself but that she can't help it. You have had this conversation with her many times over the last two years.

5. Choose a situation in your current practice where you really do not want to work with a particular person:

   • Now consider how you can protect yourself from your dislike and work constructively with the person.

   • What will you be doing differently?

Fortunately, solution focused practice does not ask you to empathise with or like the people with whom you work. All that you are expected to do is politely and curiously ask solution focused questions – although in the first scenario we would agree that Norman has forfeited the right to be near his old environment and we would look for a care home where he is unlikely to be recognised. Where we have taken a dislike to a person, we have found ourselves sticking resolutely to solution focused practice techniques – no pleasant asides, just curious questions. In these instances, we have been mildly surprised to discover that we make the most rapid progress – so maybe we shouldn't bother with pleasantries?

You wouldn't be in health and social care, however, if you didn't enjoy the work and the people you meet so another way of handling those who are annoying, frustrating or downright horrible is to make an attempt to understand their position in life, particularly the hardships they have experienced. These don't excuse their behaviour but they do help you see the person as more than just an oppressor of others, including you.

CASE EXAMPLE

James was attending a domestic violence programme following his wife leaving him after an argument where he put his arm across her throat in bed, half throttling her. She is living in a refuge and he is desperate to get her back. He has a long history of violence, dating back to when he was an enforcer in the Irish Troubles. When asked about the influence of violence on his life, he talked about the mixed emotions that went with it – excitement, power, fear and shame. He talked about how he recognised how brutalised he had become but that he was fearful for his safety if he stopped. He had moved abroad in an attempt to get away from violence. James still has to deal with his assault on his wife and the broken relationship but by putting his violence in context, it is hard not to see James as *both* victim and offender.

Similarly, in the example of Ayesha (above), it is important to understand the meaning of self-harm to a person, which is often to exert some control in a life that seems uncontrollable – and may have been for some years. Gallop and Tully (2003) cite a young woman who had been abused by her father for many years, who said that cutting gave her control over how badly she is treated now. She can decide when to cut, how deeply and when to stop. Another woman told us that seeing the blood run gave her a sense of release, whilst another said it soothed her. Alternative, less harmful strategies for attaining peace, control and comfort can be developed once the meaning of the harm is understood (for more details, see Milner and Myers 2017, ch.4).

CASE EXAMPLE

'When I go to A and E, they say straight off, "Which arm is it this time?" I feel that big. It's so embarrassing. I try not to go to hospital now but the stitching helps. It distracts me from the thoughts. Not being able to go leaves me coping with a bad patch on my own.'

PRACTICE ACTIVITIES

1. Ask a person with a tattoo (or yourself, if you have one) the following questions:

    - I've noticed you have a tattoo, would you be interested in talking about it?

    - Could you say a little about the meaning of that tattoo?

    - Does it symbolise or stand for anything in particular?

    - What led to your decision to get that tattoo?

    - Does that tattoo represent a stand for or against something?

    - Did it mark a particular transition in your life?

    - What difference does the tattoo's presence make in your life?

    - Does the tattoo suggest anything about who you are or what you might hold to be important?

    (Boucher 2003)

Adapt these questions to make them appropriate for someone who is self-harming.

2. Choose a situation in your current practice where you really do not want to work with a person:

    - List three things you can do differently that will make the work more pleasant and effective.

Allowing risk and responsibility taking

'Twenty years from now you will be more disappointed by the things that you didn't do than by the ones you did do. So throw off the bowlines. Sail away from the safe harbor. Catch the trade winds in your sails.'

(Mark Twain)

We start from the principle that people have the right to make their own decisions while minimising risk or harm to themselves or others. People want more control over their health, treatment and care, and this has led to guidance that centralises the voice of the person in this process: 'Service users should have the opportunity to make informed choices about their care and treatment in partnership with their healthcare professionals' (NICE 2011, p.8). This can create tensions for workers as people may well want to take decisions that are risky, which can make the worker vulnerable if they go along with this and things go wrong. In a litigious world, this can lead to defensive practices that seek to avoid risk and blame.

Taking this context into account, we need to find ways of supporting people to make decisions that are as informed as possible, working with them to be clear about any risks and how they can best be managed. The Supported Decision Tool produced by the Department of Health (DoH 2007, p.51) contains a good focus on the person's wishes and strengths as well as the possible risks and how these might be alleviated or managed. It includes the following questions:

- What is important to you in your life?

- What is working well?

- What isn't working so well?

- What could make it better?

- What things are difficult for you?

- Describe how they affect living your life.

- What would make things better for you?

- What is stopping you from doing what you want to do?

- Do you think there are any risks?

- Could things be done in a different way which might reduce the risks?

- Would you do things differently?

- Is the risk present wherever you live?

- What do you need to do?

- What do staff/services need to change?

- What could family/carers do?

- Who is important to you?

- What do people important to you think?

- Are there any differences of opinion between you and the people you said are important to you?

- What would help to resolve this?

- Who might be able to help?

- What could we (practitioner) do to support you?

- Agreed next steps – who will do what?

- How would you like your care plan to be changed to meet your outcomes?

- Record of any disagreements between people involved.

- Date agreed to review how you are managing.

The Mental Capacity Act 2005

This Act states that capacity is to be presumed until proven otherwise. By 'capacity' is meant the ability to comprehend information relating to a decision, to retain that information, to use and weigh it to arrive at a choice and to communicate the decision (even if only by blinking an eye). The Act obliges services to take all practical steps to support people in making their own decisions as far as is practicable, in an environment in which the person is comfortable with the aid of an expert in helping the person to express their views.

Capacity is not to be ruled out simply because a person makes an unwise decision – s/he has the right to irrational or eccentric decisions that others might judge to be not in their best interests. If capacity is judged to be lacking, services must use the least restrictive option for caring, the option that would least restrict the right to freedom of action. A person may lack capacity in regard to one matter but not to another. The incapacity may be caused by mental or physical illness, learning disability, dementia, brain damage or a toxic or confused state.

Any action taken on the person's behalf must be based on their best interest, not simply on age, appearance or assumptions based on condition or behaviour, or assumptions as to whether s/he will have quality of life without treatment. All relevant circumstances are to be considered and none is to be seen as more important than another. It cannot be assumed that a person will not recover capacity later on. Past and present wishes and feelings are to be considered, and any written statements and religious beliefs. The Act does not mean that a doctor has to continue life-sustaining treatment when it is not in the person's best interests. The burden of proof of incapacity lies with the assessing health professional, who would work with social workers, as many decisions involve considerations of care provision.

The Mental Capacity Act 2005 is relevant in working with not only those who are mentally ill but also those with dementia and those with learning disability. Developments in case law have highlighted the limitations of the Deprivation of Liberty Safeguards Code of Practice in guiding assessment making. Brindle *et al.* (2013) recommend that in order to ensure the person's best interests are served at all times, it is essential to 'make a detailed analysis of all restrictions to which the person is subject and then imaginatively consider how the care plan might be modified to minimize the effects of the restrictions' (p.83). This will require moving away from procedurally dominated assessments as Macdonald (2010) found that social workers who adopted a rights-based orientation to assessment were more likely to support older people with dementia to articulate their preferences and advocate for them to retain their chosen lifestyles.

A further important value is that of ensuring that the service user is able to use their own language, whether it be sign language or Welsh, or possibly Welsh sign language. This is to be a core component of work with older people, not an optional extra. This does not simply mean that the assessing social worker needs to be skilled in talking with people; they are also required to provide 'evidence-based written information tailored to service user needs...[which] should be culturally appropriate...accessible to people with additional needs, such as physical, sensory, or learning disabilities, and to people who do not speak or read English' (NICE 2011, p.8).

CASE EXAMPLE

Janice, a single lady of 53 years of age, was referred by a social worker with deaf people. He requested an assessment as he was concerned that she may not be capable of managing her affairs, which were being dealt with by a solicitor, and also to discuss her residential placement, as she was living in a homeless family unit.

Janice presented as a pleasant, anxious, severely deaf woman of low average intelligence. Her speech was intelligible and she was able to lip-read reasonably well in a one-to-one situation. She gave a reasonable account of her past history but was unaware of the extent of her savings, which were considerable. She had a rough idea of the amounts of money that she had in two bank accounts but had no idea how much she had in the third one. She had deposits in five different building societies, but had no idea how much she had in any of them. She was not happy with her solicitor and wished to find another one. Subsequent psychometric assessment indicated that she had a degree of mental impairment. It was recommended that her affairs should be placed in the hands of the Court of Protection.

Janice was found accommodation at a hostel. She settled well in her new accommodation. At a later date, she decided that she wanted to make a will. Her living relatives had had no contact with her for many years and she decided to bequeath her money to two charities – one for deaf people and the other for the mentally impaired. She recalled that a girl with Down's syndrome used to live next door when she was a child. (Adapted from Denmark 1994, pp.109–110)

PRACTICE ACTIVITY

Ninety-year-old Conchita has been admitted to your nursing home from hospital following a fall. She is Spanish but has lived in England for over 50 years. She has no family but had a wide circle of friends, most of whom are deceased, although two women friends are also in care homes. She has been diagnosed as suffering from dementia and needs a high level of nursing care. She is often verbally abusive (in Spanish) to staff, especially when they try to stop her wandering out of the home. She has threatened to hit them with her stick:

- How will you approach communicating with Conchita?

Carers remain entitled to their own assessments and these may well reveal conflicting and competing needs. Gridley, Brooks and Glendenning (2012) suggest that assessing the needs of the carer and cared-for person jointly is an effective way of delivering care.

PRACTICE ACTIVITY

Both in their late 70s, Bill had been caring for Peggy over a three-year period, which saw her becoming increasingly dependent following a series of strokes and Parkinson's disease. Bill then suffered a heart attack and was admitted to hospital only to discharge himself when he heard that Peggy was to be admitted to a care home. The worker provided a package of domiciliary and respite care, which met the couple's needs until Peggy broke her hip in a fall. Her mobility seriously restricted, the worker, concerned about Bill's health, again suggested admission to a home. Bill strongly resisted this plan:

> She's [worker] always asking me how I'm coping but that's only to get her into a home. I do it [caring] 'cos I want to. I do get tired but if she's at home, I won't be trotting up here [hospital] to see her. I still hurry home from the shops, I look in the room for her, even though I know she's not there. I can read her, if she gets unsettled, I know what she wants. I know what questions to ask her. Anyone else wouldn't realise this.

The Care Act 2014 says that patients have the right to make choices about their care and treatment, including decisions about their safety, even when those decisions may seem to others to be unwise:

- How would you balance Bill's rights with your concerns about his and Peggy's safety?

Workers may issue dire warnings about consequences but, as we can see in the example of Bill above, this is not a particularly effective way of engaging people. It particularly doesn't work with young adults for whom risk taking is part and parcel of growing up, particularly around the area of drink and drugs. Couzens says, 'How to talk about drugs and alcohol needs thoughtfulness. There's often this concept that everything about drugs and alcohol is negative. It's pretty hard to have an interesting conversation if everything is negative!' (1999, p.26). You can have an interesting conversation about safety and responsibility taking, however, such as:

- When you go out drinking at the weekend with your mates, how will I know that you will be all right?

- What can you do, and what can I do, to help me understand that you will be all right?

- What are the things that make you know you are going to be all right?

- Could you tell me about them? I might feel a whole lot safer about it if I knew those things.

These questions can be varied for a wide variety of risk-taking situations, such as taking responsibility for physical health (Whiting 2006) and sexual health (Myers and Milner 2007).

PRACTICE ACTIVITY

Think of a young person with whom you are working whose risky behaviour worries you; for example, a young person who puts their diabetic control at risk by neglecting to inject themselves when they are out with mates. Make a list of the questions and advice you have offered in the past. Keep only those that worked well (don't worry if none of them worked; ignoring advice is what young people do). Now, devise a set of safety questions that are appropriate to your work setting.

People who can't or won't talk

If you work with people with little or no speech, you are probably already experienced in the use of appropriate aids. Even where you don't have specialist knowledge to enable you to talk with a person who lacks speech, however, you can adapt a technique described by Iveson (1990) where you consult another family member. You simply ask them, 'If [person's name] could speak, and I were to ask her to choose someone to speak for her, who do you think she would choose?' After some discussion, agreement is usually reached on who understands the person best and can speak for them. If the person has any way at all of communicating, such as nodding, we then ask the person if the others have chosen the right person to represent them. And then we interview that person as the other.

This can get confusing in situations where the person representing the one without speech also has something to say on their own account. Here we make it clear which one of them we are speaking to by using their different names at the beginning of each question or comment we make. Where people won't speak, the worker needs to find out how they wish to communicate, and what their silence means.

CASE EXAMPLE

When I was volunteering in a low care residential home a few years ago, a lady with advanced dementia decided to tag along with my father-in-law and me. The staff regularly told me not to waste my time with her as she could no longer speak. However I took a real shine to her and had time to spend with her, so two to three times a week we either sat or walked together, arm in arm. Initially she would ask me if she knew me, with a worried look on her face. Over the course of a few months, she not only recognized my face and started greeting me with a smile, but she shared with me all sorts of things about herself, where she had grown up, how her father had the first car in her district, and other interesting details of her life. Yes, she could talk – she just needed people to take the time for her to find her words, and then for them to listen. Each time I would meet with her, I would tell her the things she had last shared with me, and she would eventually be delighted that although she had thought that there was nothing in there (pointing to her head), she still knew the things about herself, and wished others would take time to let her find her words. Her words, not mine. (Swaffer 2016, pp.144–145)

When we are meeting with people with a learning or memory difficulty, we have found it helpful in facilitating strengths-based conversation at the beginning (and throughout) the work, to use Strengths cards (https://innovativeresources.org/). This is a pack of colourful picture cards which have a particular quality written on each one; for example, patient, organised, caring and so on. The cards can be introduced in an individual session or incorporated in a family or group session whereby you ask individuals to pick those (or limit it to, say, one or two) that they think represent themselves, or ask one family member to pick for another. It is important to get a rich description of how a particular strength has been displayed. Equally, families in difficulty can struggle to see the 'good stuff', so a useful question is, 'How will you adapt to [the diminished mental or physical ability] in a way that brings out the best in you and your family?'

Talking with people with autism

People with autism give a different meaning to experiences, a meaning that people without autism often cannot understand. Therefore, people with autism respond to these experiences in a way that is likely to be found 'weird' or unusual by other people. But if you take the time to learn how people with autism give meaning to experiences, it turns out that their actions aren't illogical at all. (Mattelin and Volckaert 2017)

Remembering how people with autism process social information helps the worker communicate more effectively by:

- Keeping the topics unambiguous and concrete, using short, clear questions and going at a slow pace so that the person can process both your words and their meaning.

- Using visual images to support your conversation as these are more easily understood and less ambiguous than words.

- Organising any information you need to impart beforehand so that the agenda for the meeting is clear.

- Using social stories, anecdotes and tailor-made scenarios to help people prepare for new social situations (for more details on social stories, see Grey 2010). These should be personalised and future oriented.

- Avoiding small talk as it may be seen as a confusing digression (Mattelin and Volckaert 2017).

Key points

We consider it to be very important that we are respectful of where people start from and to join with them on their own terms, trying to understand the world from their point of view rather than filter it through our understanding. We aim to do this by:

- looking for opportunities to give people their own voice

- listening to that voice without being confused by the problem.

We need to remember that the problems are the problems; the people are not the problems. We need to be especially careful not to let a problem story represent the totality of the person by:

- Refusing to 'sum people up', remaining uncertain, open to contradictions and to possibilities.

- Speaking with people as active agents in the creation of their lives, worlds and selves.

- Avoiding assumptions that might limit their potential, such as ideas about deficit, pathology or any single label.

Our basic values include a strong belief in kindness, dignity and a constant search for each person's uniqueness.

Chapter Three

Setting Achievable Goals

In this chapter, we discuss the importance of constructing helpful and realistic goals and we describe different ways of doing this. Developing well-formed goals is a vital part of getting the best outcomes from work; however, it can also be very difficult to do this. Sometimes, people don't know what they want from the work or what their best hopes are, or their life might have been so difficult that they can't imagine it being better. Quite often, people are too ashamed or embarrassed to talk about their hopes and wishes as they have not been encouraged to see themselves as worthy of such consideration. They can also be overwhelmed by the expectations of those around them such as family and professionals, or simply not accept or recognise that there is a problem at all.

We explore various techniques to help develop goals in these difficult situations. First, we look at goal setting where people are able to express hope for the future. Later in this chapter, we look at goal setting where people feel helpless or hopeless. Central to solution focused practice is the development of hopefulness – no matter how dire the person's situation.

Forming goals

We think that it is important to have clear goals in any work with people, as, otherwise, you and they will have no way of knowing whether or not your intervention has been effective. A simple way of identifying their preferred future is by asking:

- How will you know that meeting with me will be worthwhile?

- What are your best hopes from our meeting?

- What are the things you want to bring up?

- What are your best hopes for your treatment?

- What will need to happen for you to know that our work is helpful to you?

- What things are important to your family?

- What are your best hopes for your family?

- What will other people notice is happening differently?

- What will you notice is happening differently?

We find that it is easier to measure whether you and the person have achieved your goals if you have defined them in clear, concrete behavioural changes; for example, 'I will be taking my medication as prescribed' or 'I will be calmer so that anxiety doesn't panic me.' These broad goals are then developed by asking the person further follow-up questions for detail, such as:

- What are your thoughts about the usefulness of this medication for you?

- What could you do to make sure the medication works for you?

- What do you already know about the possible side effects of this medication?

- What possible side effects would you be willing to live with?

- What is needed for you to persevere with this medication?

- How would you notice that you no longer need this medication?

- How would others notice that you no longer need this medication?

- Suppose a good friend had the same problem and was considering taking medication. What would your advice be?

- You must have a good reason for not wanting to take this medication. Please tell me more.

(Adapted from Bannink 2010)

Or you may ask what they will be doing differently when they are calm: 'Suppose I looked through a window into your house and saw you being calm. What would I see, what would you be doing? What does being calm look like?' This helps to ensure that the worker is really clear about what calm behaviour means to the person. It also helps them discuss the detail of what they will be doing when their best hopes are achieved, which increases their sense of ownership of the process. Questions can be asked about how they have managed to be calm; what it was that helped them to do this; and what personal qualities they are using to make sure they retain control over their anxiety.

Goals do not have to be modest ones; there is evidence that seemingly unachievable goals lead to more success than smaller ones. For example, a study of obese people (Avery *et al.* 2016) found that people with an ambitious dream weight goal dropped an average of 19 per cent of their body weight on a 12-month slimming course, whilst those who set a target of only 10 per cent of their body weight achieved exactly that. But, generally, you and the person will start out with the simplest, most easily achievable goal.

CASE EXAMPLE

Often, people with mental ill-health are deemed to be irrational and their responses can be dismissed as unrealistic or bizarre. Hawkes, Marsh and Wilgosh (1998) describe goal setting with a man who hears voices, using his expressed hope of becoming England's next football manager to develop ideas for how to achieve this. These ideas were actually helpful in getting back on track with his everyday life, as they required him to take his medication, behave sociably and attend for treatment, which were the first steps to becoming the England manager as well as being back in control of his life. This was not only an ethical, achievable, measurable and desirable goal, but it was also one that kept his dreams and best hopes alive. The small steps/goals took him along the path to his greater hope, allowing him to make a start. He may not reach his final goal, but his quality of life will improve enormously while trying to achieve it.

People have a tendency to describe goals negatively, such as, 'I won't be drinking to excess any more; Sharon will stop shouting at me.'

Again, it is easier to measure whether or not you have been effective if your goals are framed in terms of the *presence* or *start* of something rather than *absence* or *end* of something. For example, it is more useful to talk about the start of controlled drinking days than the end of excessive drinking days (where it is impossible to say when it will happen). A more positive goal for dealing with Sharon's shouting could be developed by asking, 'What do you want Sharon to do instead of shouting?' and 'What will you be doing differently when she is no longer shouting? Could any of this happen now?'

CASE EXAMPLE

Steve was undertaking an assessment of Jack about his sexual offending. Jack said that he was not going to do it again so Steve asked how he and the court could be certain that Jack was not going to do it again. Jack looked puzzled, then said that we couldn't because there was no way he could prove to us that he was never going to do it again. He said that he could continue not to do it forever (he hadn't repeated his offending since being caught) but there was always the suspicion that he would do it again the next day.

Steve then began to discuss with Jack what he could be doing more of that would develop confidence in everyone that he would not do it again. Jack was able to identify several actions that he needed to take that would make people believe in him, including behaving better at home, seeing his psychologist regularly, keeping his job and abiding by the restrictions placed on him by the court.

Sometimes, we simply ask, 'If this were a shop where you could buy a solution to your problem, what would you buy today?' It is possible to establish a goal even when someone cannot bring themselves to say what the problem is, perhaps due to the embarrassing or hurtful nature of the problem, which means that they are not yet ready to go into detail. Acknowledging this, we may ask, 'When everything is sorted and the problem isn't worrying you any more, what will be different?' It being possible to develop solutions without knowing what the problem is seems counterintuitive to most problem focused work where understanding the problem is seen to underpin any solution; however, questions such as, 'Can you think of a time when the problem has been a bit less of a problem?' and 'Can you remember what was happening differently then?' open up exceptions that can be used by the person to reflect on how change may be achieved.

Sometimes, workers, and their managers, confuse outputs (what services they are providing) with outcomes (what is different as a result of those services). This can lead to further confusion; for example, a man who is violent to his partner may be told that he has to go on an anger management programme. He does so but his behaviour does not change because the approach has not worked with him, so, although he has done what was asked of him (outputs), his behaviour is still deemed to be a problem (outcomes). This creates frustration for him as he is carrying the failures of a programme that was not suitable for him. Solution focused workers would view this as not having found his unique way of cooperating with us and ask him curious questions about what sort of programme would work for him – we have yet to work with a man whose goal was to continue being violent (Milner and Myers 2016).

We use the word 'instead' a great deal to help people become clearer about their goals. For example, 'He won't be going out getting drunk any more' will be developed by asking, 'When he's not going out getting drunk any more, what will he be doing instead? And what else?' When goals are defined in this way they become more imaginable and achievable. Where there are safeguarding concerns, people should also receive clear messages about exactly what needs to be different for the worker to be confident that their work is finished. This includes what small signs they will notice in their behaviour to warrant a reduction in professional concerns. Again, it helps if this is phrased in positive rather than negative terms. For example, when working with a parent whose drinking puts the children at risk of neglect, you may well set goals such as:

- The parent will book a responsible babysitter before going drinking.

- The rent payments will be up to date.

- There will be enough food in the fridge to make a healthy meal for the children.

- The parent will be up in time to get the children to school.

- The children will be clean and tidy.

- The parent will be attending school events and helping with homework.

PRACTICE ACTIVITY

Choose a safeguarding situation in your current practice and:

- List your concerns on the left-hand side of a piece of paper.

- On the right-hand side of the paper, list the constructive behaviours that concerning person will be doing differently that completely answer each concern.

- On a separate sheet, list what the vulnerable person will be doing differently that provides you with some evidence that they are safer.

It is equally important for a person to be given the opportunity to say how best professionals can support them and what needs to be different to increase the likelihood of the preferred outcome being achieved. This is about respecting people's views and making sure that we hear what they have to say. What people want is often quite straightforward: that professionals turn up on time for appointments; that there will be no hidden agendas at meetings; that professionals are clear about what needs to be different if they are to no longer need intervention; and that they won't be 'dumped' when interventions turn out not to work.

We have found that this sharing of responsibility of what everyone involved could do to achieve the best outcome has encouraged a greater collaborative relationship with families. This is the case with most people; where you are professional and respectful, they are likely to view themselves as being worthy of respect. Many of the people we work with often struggle to see themselves as of value, sometimes due to the way they have been brought up, sometimes because of the way society has treated them, sometimes because of their situation and sometimes because of their bad behaviour. We consider that even where the person has behaved in ways that have harmed others, they still deserve to be treated as human beings.

Goals do change and develop further over time, but must always be achievable, time-limited and measurable, otherwise you and the person don't really know what you are doing. More questions to aid goal setting include:

- What sort of person do you want to be?

- What can you see yourself doing when you will be doing [the goal], right here today?

- What will people notice that will be different when you are doing [the goal]?

- How might they respond differently to you?

- How do you think this will be helpful to you?

- When will be the first opportunity to do [the goal]?

- How will you know when you/I don't need to come here any more?

- How will I know that you/I don't need to come here any more?

The miracle question

De Shazer (1988, p.5) gave this name to a specific question that has been shown to work particularly well in developing goals. It is quite long and is especially useful in helping people who struggle to say what their best hopes are. We have to use caution when using the word 'miracle' as we often work with people who may well have been sexually abused and we are aware that words like 'miracle' or 'magic' can be related to the tricks abusers have used. We use words such as 'something wonderful' instead. Although it sounds formulaic, the miracle question works well because it is a curious question; you can never be sure what the answer will be. It goes like this:

Now, I want to ask you a strange question. Suppose that while you are sleeping tonight and the entire house is quiet, a miracle happened. The miracle is that the problem which brought you here is solved. However, because you are sleeping, you don't know that the miracle has happened. So when you wake up tomorrow morning, what will be different that will tell you that the miracle has happened and the problem which brought you here is solved?

This is followed by gentle prompts about new behaviours, new attitudes and new relationships, followed by, 'Is any little bit of this happening already, sometimes?' So, the miracle question helps to get a picture of the future without the problem, and the follow-up searches out small exceptions to the problem. When these are found the key question then is, 'How did you do that?' This is not only a self-compliment but it presupposes personal agency and builds up possibilities of repeating what they are able to do – at least once. With some small exceptions, a minimum of motivation and a little imagination, when we use constructive questions the possibilities are boundless and the person can get ready for change and development without analysing the problem – they can 'describe what they want without having to concern themselves with the problem and without traditional assumptions that the solution has to be connected with understanding or eliminating the problem' (de Shazer 1994, p.273).

Berg and Reuss (1998) recommend pausing for a long time after asking the question. People are not used to being asked about miracle days so it is a hard question to answer and needs a lot of thought before answering. Some workers find it is helpful for people when they ask the question in a particular way, using their voice and a sense of drama to encourage people to engage with the question.

This includes speaking slowly and softly, which gives the person some space and time to move from a focus on problems to a focus on solutions, and introducing the miracle question in a dramatic way that emphasises that it is a an unusual and strange question. The conversation is paced slowly with frequent pauses to allow the person to understand and process the question. There is a focus on the future and the use of future-oriented language, such as 'How will things be different?' and 'How will you know the miracle has happened?' When asking further questions it is useful to encourage people to think about when the problem is solved so that a solution focus is maintained, and when people fall into problem-talk then gently encourage them to look at what would be different when the miracle happens. For more details see De Jong and Berg (2007).

The above may be useful for people who have learning difficulties by taking a slower, clearer and more methodical approach; however, we find that such strategies are often helpful for everyone, whatever their label. Discussing what will be happening that is different may be the person's first opportunity to actually consider what life could be like, and rehearse this; for example, when someone responds with, 'I'll have less pain,' you will follow up with questions about what they will be doing differently when they have less pain. Managing distressing symptoms is an important goal in the short term but many people have longer-term goals that are to do with a desired lifestyle, or how to achieve an early discharge from hospital, or work on life skills (Macdonald 2011; Burns 2016). Therefore, a helpful goal will refer to some other behaviour that the person is hoping to see or do.

Goal-setting questions can include other people in the person's life as it can help to consider other perspectives to get a clearer picture of what might be achieved. A question can be asked such as, 'What would your partner notice differently about you?' of someone who is unhappy and depressed. It is possible to ask people who feel isolated and lonely to consult their pets; for example, 'What would your dog see you doing when you are feeling happier?' An answer may be very simple, but still constitute a desirable and measurable goal; for example, 'I will be smiling at the X Factor on TV' or 'I will be humming along to my music.' Where people struggle to think what would be different, remember to be patient and don't jump in with suggestions; continue with more questions, such as:

- What will you notice; what else; what else; what else?

- What will you see?

- What will be different?

- What will other people notice about you?

- Picture later in the morning: what is happening now; what else is telling you the miracle has happened?

- At work/home/other places, what is different here?

- Back at home, late afternoon, what do you notice now?

- What sort of things are you saying to yourself at the end of the day?

For unrealistic answers like 'winning the lottery', 'all my work colleagues will have been sacked' or 'I'll have absolute power', then ask:

- So, what will *you* be doing differently then?

- Can any of this happen now?

When people respond initially with 'I don't know' or silence, remain very still and quiet for a few seconds as this is likely to be the space where the person is formulating their answers. If the worker makes a verbal or physical response too soon, then this can be seen as claiming their turn to speak, which will close down this process. There are some clues to whether people are thinking about the question; for example, if they make quick eye movements up and to the right, or their eyes go slightly out of focus. Although not definitive, these do seem to indicate that people are generating new material and are promising signs that the question has had an impact. Going slowly and continuing to offer helpful follow-up questions are good practices here:

- Look puzzled and wait.

- 'It's a difficult question…'

- 'Maybe you know and don't know at the same time, that's hard to say…'

- 'Take your time and think about it, there's no rush.'

- 'Guess.'

- 'Suppose you did know, what would the answer be?'

- 'Perhaps I've not asked this question in a helpful way; how could I ask it better?'

- 'What advice would you give to a person with a similar problem to you?'

- 'Perhaps you might like to study what happens next time and see if you can spot how you did it.'

- 'Okay, so what would [name of loved one] say about it?'

Burns (2016) reminds us to be conscious of cultural and religious differences that may make it difficult for a person to answer miracle questions. For example, she suggests that it would be hard for some Christians and Muslims who believe that their situation is 'God's will' so a different perspective is needed; for example, 'What would God notice you doing differently?' (p.53).

CASE EXAMPLE

Joan feels her recovery has reached a plateau since her stroke 2 years ago. The physiotherapist feels she has unrealistic expectations regarding mobility. Joan responds to the miracle question with:

Joan: I wake up and I can turn over. I can stand up and walk on my own... I can get to the bathroom. I make breakfast.

Therapist: What else?

Joan: I'll be able to put my arms round my partner Roy. He is wonderful... He does everything.

Therapist: How will you be feeling?

Joan: Relief. I'll agree to go to the park and feed the ducks. I'll make steak and chips for him, and his favourite tomatoes with garlic.

Second session

Joan and Roy have been for a walk in the park and her friends have noticed a difference in how she is coping generally. Joan and Roy are joking, touching and comforting each other throughout the session. Roy is asked the miracle question:

Roy: We'll get up. Joan can do her thing, and then after breakfast we'll have a walk... In the forest, by the sea... There will be sunlight.

Therapist: It's interesting that you both are looking at the same thing; being together... Like a normal couple. How different is this from what you're doing already?

Joan: I watch a lot of TV. I know Roy doesn't like me doing that but I don't want to bother him. I feel guilty watching TV though.

Therapist: What would you like to feel instead?

Joan: That I deserve it. So if I do some exercises first, then I feel I deserve a rest and I can watch TV.

Roy: I saw my mother sit in front of the TV and die of cancer. I'm fearful that Joan will fill her brain with soaps...

Therapist (turning to Joan): How can you help Roy with his concerns?

Joan: I'll do some ironing, read a book, wash up, try the computer...

Therapist: Gosh! And what can Roy do to help you with your concerns?

Joan: He can show himself more self-respect. Not always put everyone else's needs first.

Roy: Yes. I know what I need to do. I need to lose weight. I've been bad tempered these last two years. Angry.

Therapist: What do you want to feel instead?

Roy: Calm. I need to do things for myself. I need to get out... Have time out.

(Burns 2016, pp.132–133)

PRACTICE ACTIVITY

As a worker, you know that you struggle with a heavy workload. This causes you anxiety, especially as you and your line manager are under pressure due to an imminent inspection. Imagine that you go home tonight, have dinner and relax, then go to bed as usual. During the night, something wonderful happens, and you are completely free from anxiety. Because you are asleep, you do not know that this is the case:

- When you go to work in the morning, what will be the first thing you notice that will tell you that anxiety has left you?
- What will your colleagues notice that is different?
- What will your line manager notice that is different?
- What will you be doing differently?
- Can any of this happen already?

Group miracle question

The miracle question can also be used with groups. Sharry *et al.* (2001, p.136) suggest asking group members to close their eyes, relax each muscle in turn and visualise a relaxing scene before asking the miracle question. Then they are asked to imagine the new solution situation in detail:

> *You are going to be surprised at all the differences and changes you notice... So what do you notice first?... What tells you the miracle has happened?... How do you feel different?... What do you notice is different about other people?... and so on.*

After the visualisation process, members discuss the differences in pairs, and then in the whole group. The advantage of this is that the solutions generated by group members are likely to have common links and this can be reinforcing when shared in the whole group. Also, hearing other people's miracles can be motivating and inspiring and encourage people to develop their own. Don't worry if the group format encourages silliness when working with young adults; it will start the group thinking and they may need time to work out their goals – as is seen in the case example below.

CASE EXAMPLE

Judith was working with a group of young women, misusing substances, and at risk of being drawn into prostitution by older 'boyfriends' who supplied drugs and drink. They had no idea what their goals for the group might be, so Judith asked the most vocal young woman the miracle question. Marie's miracle day turned out to be one where she would be not living at home, and having an endless supply of drugs and drink without having to pay for them. Rather than tell Marie that this was an unacceptable goal, Judith puzzled with Marie about how her goal would fit with her referrer's worries about the group: concerns about safety. This enabled all the young women to talk about how they did or didn't manage to keep themselves safe when they were misusing substances, and they developed a group goal around increasing safety.

Although the miracle question had yielded only one goal that was immediately useable, the young women insisted that any new group member 'do the miracle thing' and their 'keeping safe' goal broadened their individual goals, these being increasingly talked about as 'getting a life', reducing arguments with parents, handling boyfriends, and 'getting some work done so I can pass my exams'. (Milner 2004, p.15)

Nightmare question

Recovery from substance misuse is sometimes complicated by the predicament it causes some people. Reuss noticed this with so-called hardcore drinkers: 'Faced with continued drinking, which placed their jobs in jeopardy, or quitting, which placed all their friendships in jeopardy, these alcoholics did not see abstinence as a solution, but just as "another damn problem"' (Berg and Reuss 1998, p.36). Similarly, heroin use involves the person in a very busy and social day; quitting would leave the person with a large empty space. Rather than give up on what were seemingly 'hopeless cases', Reuss designed the 'nightmare question':

> *Suppose when you go to bed tonight, sometime in the middle of the night a nightmare occurs. In this nightmare, all the problems that brought you here suddenly get as bad as they possibly can get. This would be a nightmare. But this nightmare comes true. What would you notice tomorrow morning that would let you know you were living a nightmare life?*

The follow-up to the nightmare question is similar to that with the miracle question, only in reverse. When all the details of the nightmare day have been explored, experiment with bridging questions to help establish a link to possible solutions. You can ask:

- Are there times now when small pieces of this nightmare are happening?

- What is the nightmare like during those times?

- Who is most affected by the nightmare when it happens?

- And who is most interested in seeing to it that the nightmare is prevented?

- What would it take to prevent this nightmare happening?

- How confident are you that you can do what it will take?

Where couples have different nightmares, more questions are needed:

- When s/he is living his/her nightmare and you are living yours, what will you notice about each other?

- How will these nightmares destroy what you have both been working for?

The nightmare question is not to be used lightly and only after the more usual questions have been asked. Its strength is that it helps the person imagine rock bottom without actually reaching it; however, 'When you use the nightmare question we encourage you to persist with your client's perception of what his own nightmare is, instead of giving up on him as a hopeless case' (Berg and Reuss 1998, p.37). Berg and Reuss also recommend involving other significant people to counter the person who talks more about what hasn't worked than what might work and what they can do.

Variations on the miracle question

There are several variants of the miracle question, but shortened or crystal ball versions do not seem to work as well, probably because they don't encourage enough detail of what will be different. Detail is important in helping people discover solutions and ideas that they did not know they had and helps them talk themselves into change. One variation of the miracle question that we find helpful is asking the person to 'Consult your older, wiser self.' There are several ways in which this can be done; for example, Dolan (1998, p.75) asks the person to write themselves a letter from the future:

> *Suppose all the problems that brought you here have been resolved and you are living the life you want. Whilst you were busy with all these changes, you lost touch with a friend and now you are writing to her to tell her about it all. The first page of your letter describes everything that is better. Your second page begins with 'You must be wondering how this all happened. This is how I did it…' (Optional addition: It did take a lot of time but this is how I did it…)*

The follow-up questions are as described for the standard miracle question. We adapted this for younger people, calling it the 'Back to the future' question. This was inspired originally by the time machine in the Michael J. Fox film of the same name, but more recently in the UK we have used the revitalised *Dr Who* series, to which people seem to relate well:

> *Suppose today I'm still busy seeing someone else but don't like to keep you waiting around so I offer you a ride in the Tardis. You set off with the Doctor and when the doors open, you are right outside your home. You creep up to the window and look inside [adapt this bit where necessary to accommodate the*

person's mobility]. Imagine your shock when you see yourself, two years older [choose an age that is appropriate for the solution and person's capacity to think ahead]. You can tell that this person has life totally sorted out. S/he looks so happy. What is s/he doing that tells you this?

In the ensuing discussion, get as much detail as possible by asking what they are doing, who is with them, what the room looks like, whose photographs are on the wall, whose numbers are in their phone, and so on, and then you have their goal. To obtain their solution, ask:

You know how it is when someone is watching you? They get a sense of it, so you turn round and see you peering through the window [don't worry about both the 'yous', the person will know which one you are talking about]. S/he says to you, 'Oh, wow, it's me when I was in all that trouble/was so sad/felt such a failure/etc. Come in, come in.' You say, 'I haven't got long because I'm seeing this person about it all in a minute. But I must know, how did you do it?'

Most people can answer this question immediately because they have now been talking about their older, competent self at some length. For those people who struggle to answer the question, they can be invited to ask their older, wiser self for advice on comfort: 'Okay, so you can't tell me yet, but can you tell me how you got through this difficult time?' This invites the person to work out what would be comforting during the current difficulties. Additionally, because you added the word 'yet' in this question, you are presupposing that the person will be able to answer the question at some time in the future (for ideas on how people can comfort themselves, see Milner and Myers 2017, part 4).

Where people living with dementia or, indeed, any cognitive impairment are not able to tell us how they wish to receive care, Baker (2015) suggests that you research a person's documented preferences when they *did* have capacity. We see this as a sort of 'consulting your younger capable self' exercise. This involves talking with relatives to collect information about the person's life story through the construction of portable memory boxes, digital frames that provide a continuous stream of memories (and which the person does not need to hold) and A4 life story summaries. This information highlights the person's preferences about care so that they are not given food they do not like, feel uncomfortable, are given a shower when they would prefer a bath, can choose their own clothing, wear make-up and so on.

Goldsmith (2015a) makes the point that there is a tendency to dress people who need a high level of care in loose clothing as this makes it easier to assist that person. She goes on to say:

> As a person who has never owned a pair of tracksuit bottoms, I would find it incredibly confusing to suddenly be dressed in these because it was easier for somebody else. Not only would I try to remove them, it would have an impact on my well-being and sense of identity. (p.82)

Goldsmith also recommends that the carer be proactive in analysing pain, which often goes untreated in older people living with dementia: 'Dementia does not supersede existing conditions, and therefore pain relief can have a huge impact on the course of the disease' (2015b, p.173).

PRACTICE ACTIVITY

John is a resident in a home for elderly people. Staff report that he is disruptive in the dining room and keeps sliding down his chair. He pushes his food around and often needs feeding. He calls out constantly and is a nuisance to other residents in the dining room. He has lost some weight because sometimes he refuses to eat.

An interview with John's son provides the following information. Driving had been a large part of John's working life and the day he received a letter saying that his licence was being taken away upset him deeply. He phoned his son, who went over and found him on the floor having suffered a stroke. John tried to go home after being in hospital, but this proved difficult with his mobility problems. He was using a Zimmer frame but had lots of small strokes.

His son says that John is very strong-willed and determined, a very loving and caring father who loved football. He isn't one for mixing socially; he doesn't like being in big crowds. He was not a big drinker but if he did go to the pub, he would generally go with one person and sit in a corner. He enjoys the company of two to three people and he used to like listening to what was going on around him. He also likes listening to music.

John loves a cooked breakfast. He will eat it at any time of the day but needs help cutting it up into small pieces. He doesn't like chicken at all, nor curries and stews, but likes very thinly sliced beef and ham. He loves corned beef sandwiches and would often have a slice of corned beef, mashed potato and fried egg. He has become very sweet-toothed over the past few years and likes two to three sugars in his tea. He also likes to have ketchup on all his main meals. He would never eat pudding before.

- List your concerns about, and goals for, John in the above example.
- Utilising the information above, develop staff goals for helping John with his difficulties.
- Prepare a care plan which addresses these.

(Adapted from Baker 2015, p.68. For two examples of a care plan using life story work, see Baker 2015, pp.68–72)

Although the miracle question is a key element of solution focused practice in the US, many UK practitioners find it too formulaic (Walsh 2010). BRIEF (www.brieftherapy.org.uk) have found that asking a person what their best hopes are works as well as the miracle question. Macdonald (2011, p.15) provides a list of key questions for goal setting:

- What will it be like when the problem is solved?
- What will you be doing instead?
- When that happens, what difference will it make?
- How will others know that things are better?
- Who will notice first? And then who?
- What else will be different?
- What else?
- What else?

People with learning difficulties

Musker (2007) notes that the medical profession has focused on the negative side of the condition of a person with learning disabilities as their training is about identifying deficits, and that the effect for carers is that 'they see a health care profession preoccupied with what their child cannot and will not be able to do. This can be disheartening and depressing for parents and carers' (p.78). The expectations of people with learning disabilities are consequently often low, and, indeed, self-fulfilling (low expectations lead to low achievements, which, in turn, reinforce low expectations). Solution focused practice can provide opportunities to enable the person to develop their potential, sometimes by changing the expectations of those around the person.

Goal setting tends not to use the miracle question very often, possibly because people with learning difficulties can be very literal and struggle with abstract concepts and imagined futures (Lloyd, Macdonald and Wilson 2016), although it has been used successfully with people with autism spectrum disorder (Bliss and Edmonds 2007; Mattelin and Volckaert 2017). Alternatives such as, 'What are you wishing for?' and 'What will you be doing on a really good day?' are asked instead (Roeden *et al.* 2009).

When we start work with someone with learning difficulties, carers often tell us that the person doesn't concentrate well. We generally find that people with learning difficulties can concentrate for 30 to 40 minutes as long as we remember to go at a suitable pace, use appropriate materials and make it fun. People with learning difficulties do not function at all well when they are stressed, so we allow 10 minutes of settling-down time. Depending on the form the anxiety takes, this could consist of allowing silly behaviour, simply getting out our materials and talking about them in a neutral sort of way, or asking the person to undertake a simple task, such as taking care of our coat. The basic principle is to reduce the speed of everything by:

- Talking more slowly and repeating or rephrasing important points several times.

- Using pictures or symbols to explain complex concepts such as thoughts and emotions.

- Explaining ourselves through written or drawn materials as many people with learning difficulties find this method of communicating less threatening than face-to-face conversations.

- Recognising that it takes time to learn new behaviours so repeating short chunks of information several times and in fresh ways. Charts and stickers act as useful visual reminders.

- Helping the person understand new situations by keeping changes to the minimum.

- Providing opportunities to practise newly learned behaviours.

Berg and Steiner (2003) explain how cartooning makes it easier for a person with learning difficulties to develop a clear vision and sense of control over future events. Here, a large sheet of paper is divided into six squares and the person is invited to draw the problem in the first square, how they would rather be in the second, a 'mighty helper' in the third, what a slip back might look like in the fourth, how it is handled in the fifth, and how success will be celebrated in the sixth. We would not expect the person to complete all six squares in one session; as we say earlier, we would go slowly, taking one square at a time. Indeed, sometimes, the person finds their goal after the first two squares are completed and discussed.

When talking with the person about how they would rather be (square two), you will often find that their concerns are not long term; they want to be able to cope better with today and, sometimes, tomorrow. Where the person has some writing skills, we do joint story writing. For example, we will write or dictate the first line of a story about the person sometime in the future and then invite them to write the next line and so on. This not only reveals goals but often yields a solution, too. It is a particularly useful way of developing safety goals with vulnerable people as you can steer the story in the direction of dangerous situations from which the person then has to escape.

Carers have been found to overestimate the ability of people with learning difficulties to understand sexual safety issues (Banat, Summers and Pring 2002). In safety situations, we ask the person to choose a name for a person who is *similar but different* to themselves as they will find it easier to develop a story that is not directly about themselves. Sometimes, we use several techniques over a few discussions with the person before a clear goal is agreed.

CASE EXAMPLE

Gavin is a young man with learning difficulties. His mother does not let him go out alone as he has been going off with strangers and has started exhibiting inappropriate sexual behaviour.

Gavin is frustrated at being indoors and is becoming aggressive. As his family have recently moved to a different town, it will be some time before Gavin can be found a place on a training course. Gavin has chosen the name Phil for his safety story, which is translated below – with added spelling and punctuation. Phil's sentences are in a different font in bold; Judith's are in plain script.

Phil was playing on the road. This bad man came up to him. He asked Phil to show him where the pub was. This man had a nice smile so Phil did not know that he was a bad man. **Phil said no because he knew not to go with strangers.** The man smiled again, 'Go on,' he said, 'show me where the pub is and I'll give you a fiver.' **Phil said okay and went to the pub with the man**. 'Oh dear,' said the man, 'I've just remembered, all my money is at home. Jump in my car and we will get your fiver.' **Phil gets in the car with the man and the man drives off** but he doesn't go to his house. He drives out onto a lonely hill. The man isn't smiling any more. **Phil is getting very worried. He doesn't know where he is. He thinks his mum would be worrying about him. 'Give me the fiver and drive me home.'** The man stops the car, 'Stop moaning and earn your fiver,' he says. 'Take your trousers down.' **Phil got out of the car. Phil has run away as fast as he could. The bad man was set to chase him.** Phil ran and ran and ran till he found some walkers [unreadable]. **'Please, please help me.' So they take me home on the bus to his mum. His mum gave everyone [unreadable] and then she rang the police about the bad man.** Phil never got the fiver. **Phil knows not to get into cars for a fiver**.

The Mencap report *Death by Indifference* (2007) found that hospital care for people with learning difficulty can be poor, but communication and continuity of care can be much improved when a traffic lights system is used. This is a simple, colourful form which identifies important 'must know' information, including how to communicate with the person, their mental capacity, how to recognise pain and offer comfort, and their likes and dislikes (for more information, see Michael and Richardson 2008).

People with a learning difficulty or dementia are often unable to say when they are in pain so a team monitoring system is needed when analgesia is given: 'it is critical that all involved know about the pain relief given and that this is constantly evaluated' (Kerr 2007, p.110).

People with complex physical needs

However disabled a person is, they can, and should, be helped to take appropriate responsibility for their own health and make informed choices and decisions about their health and well-being (DoH 2004). The National Service Framework also wants to see professionals listening carefully and attempting to see the world from their perspective (DoH 2005). Research informs us that a diagnosis of a long-term health condition can have a devastating effect on people's emotional well-being (Forshaw 2002) and that 20 to 25 per cent of people in this situation experience significant anxiety and depression. This, in turn, makes their rehabilitation and quality of life more problematic (White 2001). The NHS guidance (NICE 2009) in the UK recommends short-term interventions such as solution focused practice for those with long-term conditions, supported by evidence that improving someone's optimism lowers anxiety and depression whilst increasing physical, social and psychological well-being (Dennison, Moss-Morris and Chalder 2009).

Carr, Smith and Simm (2014) evaluated the impact of solution focused practice with people with long-term conditions and found that people felt:

- more empowered and in control of their difficulties

- more able to use their existing skills in new ways to better manage their illness

- increased hopefulness for the future

- good communication between the person and the worker.

In their research, the solution focused worker asked people about their wider goals in life, not simply focusing on their difficulties, and this engendered feelings of hopefulness and also reflection on what was important in their life: 'I think it gave me, unconsciously, the thought that "…I'm planning something in the future." So at the time plans for in the future was quite a good thing to do, cos it gave you a more positive thing' (Carr *et al.* 2014, p.388). Focusing on goals generates a sense of optimism and an expectation of change, rather than viewing the problem as fixed, intransigent and therefore hopeless. Reiter (2010) outlines how regularly reviewing progress towards the goals keeps people motivated, enthused and able to recognise their strengths. This is particularly important in work with people who become distressed when their condition seems to 'plateau'.

A good way to start goal setting with people is to look at anything that is already going well and agree a goal of keeping these things going and building on these. Recognising that people are already achieving some things helps to create an atmosphere of optimism and also provides material to build on. This is especially important when you are working out goals with people who don't want to talk to you for one reason or another. Where people do not consider that they have a problem, it is still important to listen to what is significant to them. People usually have good reasons for not wanting to talk to you – embarrassment, fear of consequences, possibility of losing face, despair, an episode of paranoia, and so on – but providing a space for them makes them feel respected so they may become more motivated to engage in the work. This space allows you to discover the person's own way of cooperating with you.

Whilst it is always preferable to keep your work as simple, brief and least intrusive as possible, sometimes more creativity is needed in helping people set goals. Below we outline some of the questions we have devised or borrowed for situations where people are overcome by helplessness or hopelessness. Before reading these, test out your own creativity and other skills you have developed in working with people so that these can be used to devise your own questions for effective goal setting.

PRACTICE ACTIVITY

- Make a list of all your best skills (be specific but not modest).
- How do these help you to be helpful to the people you work with?
- Choose one of these skills:
- How can you enhance this skill to make it a bit more effective?
- What would you have to do?
- When can you do it by?
- How would the people you are working with know that you are doing it better?

People who can see no future for themselves

Where people are able to express hope for the future, you can begin to work out an achievable, measurable goal; but many people find it very difficult on a first meeting with you to even begin to think about their best hopes. Some people are so depressed that they actually tell you they have no hope at all, hopelessness being their main problem. Or they are shocked on hearing that their condition is terminal, or chronic. Many people in constant pain feel that they have been given up on (Dargan *et al.* 2014; Simm *et al.* 2014). On the other hand, someone who is drinking too much and probably only has come to see you as a very last resort – probably because their partner or their employer or their doctor told them they had to come or there would be serious consequences – tend to be more concerned about what they may lose than what in actual fact they may gain by becoming a non-drinker. And some people who are in the middle of a psychotic episode may well have best hopes that seem very strange to you; for example, they may ask you to set up a block on the radio, which they are convinced is sending messages into their head. Some people with eating difficulties may have best hopes actually to be even thinner than they already are – obviously, an unethical goal.

PRACTICE ACTIVITY

Think of a person you are working with who seems utterly despairing and hopeless.

- How confident are you that you know what is really important to them in their life?

- How can you find out more about what matters to them?

- What questions would you ask that would be helpful for the person?

Someone who is struggling with depression and/or trauma may be so overwhelmed with how things are right now that they find it difficult to think what life could be like. As an alternative, enquiries can be made into how they are coping, how they are managing to get up in the morning when they are experiencing so much pain and anguish. Whilst it would be insensitive, and ineffective, to press someone for a goal in these circumstances, it is possible to hint that the future may be easier by adding a little hopefulness to coping questions, such as:

- That must be scary/terrible/worrying [then add] *at the moment* or *at this time.*

- Have you ever felt like this before? How did you get over it *last time?*

- So, you've not been able to beat…*so far?*

- How have you stopped things getting worse?

- How are you managing to carry on *despite…*?

- But you still managed to get to work; how did you find this determination?

Talking with people who are thinking about killing themselves

Hawkes *et al.* (1998, p.103) maintain that suicidal people have a specific deficit in problem-solving skills. It is this difficulty in generating alternative solutions to their problems that solution focused questions help to redress. They say that if you think of suicide as one attempted solution to a problem – but only one of many – you reduce blame for the person and value the difficult nature of their situation. You can invite them to wonder if this is the only valid solution. Asking about suicide does not put the idea into a person's head (Gallop and Stamina 2003); instead, it saves the person having to explain the seriousness of the situation and opens up discussion about alternative solutions to the problem.

Thus, an initial answer to the miracle question may be, 'I'd be dead.' This answer indicates the seriousness of the situation but then you would ask, 'How would that help?' This may produce the answer, 'My money worries would be gone, I'd have some peace, I'd be less of a burden, my family would be off my back,' and so on. Expanding these statements with, 'How could you tell this was happening?' 'What will be the first sign that you are feeling more peaceful?' 'What else would help you to do to get some rest rather than harm yourself?' and so on, begins to help the person see what they really want to be different, which may have nothing to do with death.

Questions for people who are feeling suicidal

- This option seems very hard on you, how do you deserve that?

- Did the overdose help?

- What could you do instead that will be easier on you?

- You must have a good reason for your hurting yourself…?

- Supposing in six months or so, you have to look back and see this meeting as something that turned out to be for the best, how would you know?

- If 0 is not at all and 100 is completely, how interested in the future are you?

Henden (2008) has developed these questions further:

- Tell me about a time in the last week when you felt least suicidal?

- Before you were feeling as you do at the moment, what did you do in the day that interested you?

- What has stopped you taking your life up to this point?

- On a scale of 1–10, how suicidal do you feel right now? How suicidal were you before you decided to seek help? What would you be doing/thinking/feeling that would be half a point higher?

- What have you done in the last couple of weeks that has made a difference to this terrible situation you are in?

- On a scale of 1–10, how determined are you to give other options (other than suicide) a try first?

- What would happen in this session for you to think it was worthwhile coming?

- Let's suppose you went for the last resort option and actually died. You are at your own funeral as a spirit, looking down from about ten feet at the mourners below. What might you be thinking about another option you could have tried first? Which of the mourners would be most upset? What advice would they have wanted to give you about other options?

- When was the last time before this current time that you thought of ending it all? What did you do then that made a difference and enabled you to pull yourself back?

- Let us suppose for one minute that you decide not to go for this option and you live to a ripe old age. You are looking back on your life as a person who survived this dark period and lived a purposeful and meaningful life. What would your life have been like? What sorts of things would you have done? What new people would you have known? What sort of places might you have visited? What sort of holidays would you have had? What other challenges in life might you have had to resolve? How would you have allocated time in your retirement? Where might you have seen the best sunrises and sunsets?

• Suppose you decided not to go ahead with this last resort option and you are much older and wiser than you are now. What advice would you give to you now to solve this problem/get through this time of difficulty?

Adapted from Henen 2008

Hawkes *et al.* (1998) make the important point that the solution focused approach gives the person permission to feel as bad as they do. They say:

It is not our role to dissuade them from the intensity of their feelings, only to help them find a different way of coping with these feelings. By giving permission to feel bad over traumatic life events, you humanize these feelings, introduce the idea that they may be universal and that anyone could feel as bad, given the same circumstances. (p.105)

Hawkes *et al.* (1998, p.105) suggest empowering questions such as:

• This must be an unbelievable experience for you, a nightmare. Knowing yourself as you do, what have you learned about yourself that has allowed you to get this far with the problem?

• How come you got here to see me today? How come you have held on? How have you resisted it so far?

• Does it surprise you that you have been this strong, that even given this you are still around? What about others in your life, would they have known that you were as strong as this?

They would also be curious about what the person has learned about themselves that has enabled them to resist giving into these urges so far. As Furman and Ahola say, 'traumatic experiences can be a source of learning as well as a source of distress' (1992, p.37). Hawkes *et al.*

(1998, p.62) also recommend that timeframes be considered, with questions such as: 'Is this something that will take more time to solve? Are you being hard on yourself, expecting yourself to feel very different than this?'

PRACTICE ACTIVITY

Peter has suffered from auditory hallucinations and delusions of varying intensity and content for many years, with occasional hospital inpatient treatment. He's been living independently for some years now and holding down a full-time job. Peter has volunteered to take part in a demonstration interview with a staff member of the School of Nursing. The aim of the interview was to demonstrate interview techniques and it was conducted in an interview room with students observing through a one-way mirror in an adjacent room. Peter spoke of his auditory hallucinations and his delusions. None of this was new to the interviewer until Peter stated that he believed that this year at Easter (about four weeks away) he would die. Peter explained that as he is the reincarnation of Jesus Christ and is now 33, and Christ died at Easter at the age of 33, then God will take his life at Easter. When asked what would happen if God didn't take his life at Easter, Peter replied that this would be a sign to him that he would have to take his own life. (Adapted from Walsh and Moss 2007, pp.116–117)

- Devise three questions that you can ask Peter to show that you understand how serious his problem is but also challenge his suicidal thoughts.

Hint: Walsh and Moss (2007) suggest that seeing problems as puzzles helps patients and nurses to work in a more creative and positive way. Puzzles have a different focus to problems and require people to think in a different way. Puzzles are shared. Puzzles imply solutions, creativity and a different way of looking at things to solve.

Working with people who self-harm

It can be difficult to set goals in other forms of self-harm, such as eating difficulty, which is seen as desirable by many people. As the model, Kate Moss, famously remarked, 'Nothing tastes as good as skinny feels' (Costello 2009). Equally, cutting can confer some status on the person amongst their peer group and, sometimes, a whole group of friends will decide to start cutting. Anything to do with body image is always going to be affected by media images, especially being thin, but it is worth remembering that people do like to decorate their skin. Children have always enjoyed putting transfers on their arms and now aspire to proper tattoos like their football and pop star heroes. This means that someone can be feeling both hopeless and competent when they are making cuts on their arm.

Selekman (2002) recommends asking people to invite a famous guest of their choice to act as their consultant. Having chosen their guest consultant, the person is then asked what advice their consultant would give them. Obviously, the famous guest cannot advise the person to do more harmful things, so this is one way of reducing the impact of media messages. Many of the questions for people who are feeling suicidal are helpful in working with self-harm but it is important to understand the meaning of harm to the person as this is often a way in which they feel in control of their lives. Removing one harmful behaviour may simply kick off another.

CASE EXAMPLE

Ruth had dropped out of college and her self-harming behaviour had escalated alarmingly. Although the medication she was taking obscured her voices, this did nothing to reduce the effect of the hostile voices on her self-esteem. When encouraged to talk about her voices, it emerged that she was hearing all the obscenely derogatory things her father had said over many years. The worker explored how he got into her head and what it felt like. Ruth described it as, 'a sort of octopus; it's inside my head and it's wrapped round my neck'.

They explored which 'tentacle' would be the easiest to chop off first, her self-harming being so entwined by 'the octopus' that, if she managed to stop cutting herself, she would revert to some other method of self-harm; Ruth had a very large self-harming repertoire. She decided to begin with a small goal, with the most damaging message the voice delivered, being told that she was 'a f...ing fat elephant'. Although working on eating management is probably the most difficult place to start for a woman with such significant difficulties, it was important to accept that this is where she wanted to make her first effort so an experiment was proposed: she was to study her eating behaviour and watch for the 'full sign'. She was not to attempt to stop gorging at this point, she was just to see if a 'full feeling' ever happened. Ruth was sure that she had never had such a feeling but agreed to try the experiment, which was supported by a self-pampering programme. To her surprise, she did identify several occasions when she felt 'full' and, as she was under no pressure not to eat, managed not to overeat at some of these points. This was only a tiny success in the overall scheme of her desired weight loss of many stones but it provided a starting point. After six sessions, she stopped the medication and returned to college.

Following on from her tiny successes with her eating difficulties, Ruth has been able to realise that her successes are attributable to herself and this has had an effect on her response to the voices; she now sees them as inconvenient, annoying background noise. She is also beginning to lose weight. She ascribes this to a realisation that negative thoughts weigh heavier than positive ones.

PRACTICE ACTIVITY

- If 0 is not at all and 10 is completely satisfied, how do you feel about how you look?

- If 0 is not at all and 10 is all the time, how much time you spend thinking about, or discussing with friends and colleagues, how best you can manage your fitness?

- If 0 is never and 10 is every other month, how often have you started a new diet?

If you have answered these questions honestly, you are unlikely to have low scores as healthy eating and dieting is extensively promoted in social media. But for people with eating difficulties, dieting can be fatal. Jacob (2001) says that food is a wolf in sheep's clothing: we need food to live but it can also be the enemy from which there is no escape. This makes people with eating difficulties feel helpless.

CASE EXAMPLE

Mary came home from the office Christmas party with a large slice of cream cake: 'Every time I open the fridge door, it's sat there saying, "Eat me, eat me." So, I ate half of it. Now, every time I go to the fridge, it's sat there, laughing at me.'

Goal setting with people with severe weight loss is particularly difficult as chaotic eating patterns make for chaotic thinking processes, so it is necessary to keep conversations simple. Jacob (2001) sees under-eating as a jealous liar that says, 'Stay with me, I'll keep you safe,' but this is no more than a comfort blanket is to a child; one that gets dirtier and smellier from being dragged along the floor but resists being thrown away.

It is important to ask the person questions about their goals and accept that they may wish to start off very small, indeed. The reply might be, 'I'll be able to eat a meal.' The next question would be, 'Once, or more often?' going on to check out the required period of time; and whether it means eating and keeping it down. People are often quite vague in their goals and say things like they would like to 'feel better about eating' or 'have more energy'. So, here, you continue to tease out what would be different that indicates that these goals had been reached. For example, a common goal is not to be worried about food any more, not to have it hanging over the person 24 hours a day, so you will need to ask what the person would be doing with their thoughts when they weren't using them up worrying about food. These conversations can be quite light and imaginative and people can surprise themselves with their own ideas.

Like so many other difficulties for which people seek help, eating difficulties are often influenced by relationships. Selekman (1997) gives an example of a mother worried about her son's overeating because his father was obese and died of a heart attack. The boy felt that his mother's nagging led to his 'pigging out' all the more, leaving him feeling quite defeated and distressed. Selekman spent some time with the boy visualising the future without overeating and set him a task: he secretly asked the boy to pretend to comply with his mother's wishes on eating over the next week and he – also secretly – asked the mother to 'do something different', with a view to disrupting the pattern of arguments. At the next session, the boy had created several exceptions, which were built upon.

Jacob (2001) asks people with eating disorders, 'Tell me what is useful about it' and 'What does it enable you to do differently?' Acknowledging that some problems have advantages as well as disadvantages is useful where people are extremely pessimistic, especially when followed up with, 'How can you keep the advantages but get rid of the disadvantages?' Where the person is unable to respond to any of the questions above, we have found that asking them to 'take a small step in a direction that will be good for them' and come back and tell us when they have done this is helpful in removing the misery block that is preventing them working out a goal for themselves.

Some people seem so immersed in the details of their misery that they can talk about little else, and this can be compounded for those who have experienced problem-oriented interventions. Poring over the problem does tend to lead to a problem-saturated situation (White 1995). This becomes isolating as friends who initially offer support become bored with the same problem description and irritated at their advice not being taken. In these situations, we acknowledge the extent of the person's difficulties and then make it clear that we will talk about different things from now on:

- [Looking back at our notes] Yes, I've got that. You told me that already.

- [The misery tale continues] Yes, I've got that. You told me that already.

- [The misery tale continues] We've spent a lot of time looking at the awful situation you are in. I'm wondering how useful this is? I'm thinking that it's a bit like trying to clear out a cupboard and then putting everything back, instead of sorting what needs to stay, what needs mending and what needs throwing away. So, I wondered if you'd mind if we shut the door of the misery cupboard for a while and looked in the happiness cupboard instead? What might we find in that cupboard?

- [If more than one thing is suggested] Tell me more about that happiness. How can you start to get more of it?

- [If the cupboard is pretty empty] It looks like we'll have to go shopping for some happiness. What would you like to buy first?

Talking with people who are terminally ill

Where someone is receiving palliative care for a terminal illness, the quality of the remaining time is vital, so establishing the person's goals is a matter of urgency. White (2002, personal communication) says that the ideas *miracle* and *death* seem to be at odds, but he hasn't found it a difficulty. People's goals will vary. Many reject the option to prolong their life by invasive treatment, choosing death instead; although, as White comments, this is simply life of a different kind where they can share their thoughts about dying – not just the probability of death but the many questions that follow; live as full and normal a life as possible; and participate in the process of dying. In other words, have a say whether treatment continues or not and whether to die in hospital, at home or in a hospice.

Other people may wish not to speak about it. This is not necessarily 'denial'; Bray and Groves (2007) cite the example of a woman who only spoke of her terminal cancer as 'white spots'. This was her strategy to follow her optimistic nature and not depress her son. She had previously discussed her terminal condition with a friend and grieved at that point. 'All this points to individuals having very different views of what counts as a good death and similarly many variations in the process of dying' (Scragg 2012, p.140).

The goals of the dying person will change as they do in other circumstances, so some questions could include:

- Suppose you look back after you die and you are pleased with how you have lived, what will you be pleased about?

- Suppose you are looking back after [your relative] dies and you are pleased with how you have done things, feeling you have done the right things by [your relative], what will you be pleased about?

- In here [hospice, hospital, etc.], how have you managed to keep going? What have you kept doing that you would normally be doing outside? Have you surprised yourself with how you've dealt with it? How will you know when you are dealing with it even better?

- What ideas do you have about what comes after this life?

- How will things look better for you when you have worked out what it will look like?

- How do you want your life to be between now and [next week, next month, etc.]?

- What are your best achievements?

- What hopes do you still have?

- What do you best want to be remembered for?

- What small changes in living will make a big difference for you?

Where a person is unable to speak, you can still establish a goal by consulting with their family about what sort of person their relative is. This is like the life story method described earlier but focusing particularly on what sort of person the relative has always been, what their qualities are, what ideas they have always expressed about terminal illness. This can be complicated as it is not unusual for a dying person's relatives to have different goals for them, although the question about feeling you have done the right thing by your relative would have been helpful in the case example below.

CASE EXAMPLE

Mrs Patel suffered a major stroke from which she has not recovered well. She requires constant nursing care. She is no longer able to speak or swallow so it has been suggested that she is fitted with a feeding tube in her stomach. Her elder daughter, Rani, is against this as she thinks her mother would be tortured by it. Her younger daughter, Samira, wants the procedure to go ahead as she sees it as a matter of life and death. The sisters are at total loggerheads over this.

Palliative carers say that they want full knowledge, open and frank discussion, and continuity of medical personnel who know that patient's needs and wishes (Staton, Shuy and Byrock 2001).

PRACTICE ACTIVITY

- What do you value most in life?

- What makes life worth living?

- What will be most important to you when you are dying?

- If you were to die soon, what would be left undone in your life?

(Adapted from Norlander and McSteen 2001, p.5)

It seems odd to us that some old people's goal is to die, having lived long enough, even though they are not near to death. Stern (2011) held extended conversations with elderly people who had reached 100 about their wishes and hopes. Although we tend to celebrate when a person reaches their centenary, it transpires that it can take a lot of getting used to, which, combined with worries about how dying will be, created anxiety for these centenarians.

CASE EXAMPLE

Sarah said 'it is a hardship' not to know when and how it would happen. 'It is awkward waiting to die. Everything is an effort. My time is dragging out. I am ready to go. ... Will I be on the toilet and then suddenly fall down? I hope that it will happen when I'm in bed and asleep.' The thought of reaching 103 was not a comforting one; in fact, it filled her with dread. She lamented, 'Young people die, why can't I? It would be kinder; the sooner the better.' At one stage, Sarah thought that her 'time had come'. She said 'I made myself up and lay in bed in the middle so I would look good when they found me. In the morning when I woke up, I was very disappointed. I thought that I was ready to go.' (Stern 2011, p.61)

PRACTICE ACTIVITY

Make a list of five solution focused questions that you could use to help Sarah develop a goal for living well.

Talking with people with unachievable goals

We have previously mentioned the importance of goals being achievable; however, people can choose a preferred future that is out of their control and therefore unachievable. Such an example may be someone opting for a goal of moving back in with their parents after having a violent psychotic episode and being ejected to live in sheltered accommodation. Instead of negotiating the goal, an alternative form of enquiry could be, 'I can understand that you want to move back in, but if this was something that didn't happen, how do you think you would manage/cope? What is your fall-back plan? What could the workers here do that would make the changes easier for you?'

Similar coping questions are also helpful to explore when someone has been bereaved and states that their goal would be for this person to be alive again; for example, 'Supposing [name of the person who has died] is looking down from heaven right now. S/he's going to be pretty worried about you. What advice would s/he give you for handling this problem right now?' It is also important to understand what is missed as well as the person. After a bereavement, carers often feel at a loose end, not just for the loss of a loved one but for the loss of a caring role that had mutual benefits.

PRACTICE ACTIVITY

A year after the death of his mother and partner, Kenneth was disappointed that he didn't feel any better. He was frustrated by people telling him he was suffering from an 'empty nest' syndrome. He explained that he was not grieving because he no longer had anyone to care for but for his loss of the balance between his competence and vulnerability: 'I propped them up physically, but they propped me up emotionally.'

- Make a list of at least five solution focused questions you could ask Kenneth that would help him set an achievable goal.

Where someone is living with difficulties that have to be coped with, your goal-setting questions need to take account of how you will be able to encourage hope and acknowledge the pain and fear that accompanies such difficulties. Some useful questions include:

- Each day, I'd like you to do one small thing that is good for you. We'll talk about what difference it makes.

- Each day, notice what else you do that is good for you, so we can talk about it.

- Could you keep track of the good choices you make so we can talk about them?

- As you are not yet able to defeat the problem, what can you do to stop it growing, or to make it wait (so you will be taking a little control back for yourself)? What would be the smallest step you could take?

- Perhaps you could pretend you have a future and notice the difference, so we can talk about it. What will you be doing instead of what you do now?

- What can you do that will be kind to yourself and hard on the problem? What will you be doing, or feeling, differently?

- Problems try to control us, so maybe you could confuse the problem by taking some control of your own thoughts? Think up some things to say to yourself that will help you to stand up to the problem and its lies. I'll be interested in what you come up with.

PRACTICE ACTIVITY

When Kate was diagnosed with younger onset dementia at the age of 47 she said 'being told I had dementia really was a pseudo death, and with death comes grief. You really do not have a choice. ... The sense of emptiness in your own life and on occasion towards your friends is off-putting to them, and unbearable to you. Life sometimes seems void' (Swaffer 2016, pp.111–112)

- Adapt three of the coping questions above that could be used with a person with difficulties of the magnitude of Kate's.

Key points

- A significant principle of solution focused practice is that the goal(s) of the work is decided by the person. It is the skill of the worker to support people in constructing their goals in such a way that there is a clear description of what will be different when their problems are eradicated or of less significance in their lives.

- It is important that goals are established as early as possible so that both the person and the worker have a collaborative understanding of the direction of the work. It is of equal importance that the goals are realistic and measurable. The SMART approach is useful here (Specific, Measurable, Achievable, Realistic, Time-bound). Unrealistic goals can create a situation of failure and if they are not measurable, how will you know when your support is no longer required? It is also helpful to begin this process by noticing those things that are already going well and developing and building on this with the inclusion of the desired new behaviours.

- A basic way to develop goals is to use the miracle question. This presents a future-oriented context, which invites the person to imagine what life could look like without the problem and thus identify their hopes for the work. The miracle question can also be applied within a group situation. Any future-oriented questions will assist in the formation of sound goals, however.

- Sometimes, people can struggle to describe what would be different from their perspective, but asking them from the perspective of a third party, 'What would be the first thing your partner would notice that would be different?' can often spur them on.

- A final issue to take into consideration is the possibility of goals changing during the course of the work. This may be due to the person gaining a clearer understanding of what would be most helpful for them to explore or to an initial goal having been achieved and within this process there is a realisation that it would be beneficial for a further issue to be discussed to enable them to move forward.

Chapter Four

Finding Exceptions to Problems

This chapter introduces the practice principle of finding exceptions to difficulties. Locating, and recognising, times when people have managed their behaviour in a way that is helpful and beneficial to them and others is an empowering and uplifting experience which helps engage people in a change process. There is further discussion on the importance of language: how we talk about problems; the recognition of strengths; and helping people begin to see themselves as separate from their difficulties. Techniques that support this process are also described.

Finding exceptions

Most problems have exceptions, so, once goals are agreed, the next step is to direct the conversation around exploring those times when the person's goals have happened and/or the problems they have experienced have not happened, or happened less. Focusing on those times, *the exceptions*, provides the person with an opportunity to realise that there have been better times; that they have the required skills and strengths to tackle their problems; that there are times when they are in control. Furthermore, it reinforces the assumption, mentioned in earlier chapters, that people are experts in their own lives who are equipped with the knowledge necessary for finding ways of moving forward. Because they are accustomed to being told what to do about their problems (not that they necessarily act on this advice), they are unused to being asked about their own solutions so they can struggle to locate this information. This is where the support and skill of the worker is required.

Solution focused practice recognises that there are times when the problem, however entrenched, could have happened but didn't; identifying those times will therefore also identify each person's unique solution. If you think about something you have tried to give up – smoking or chocolate, for example – there will have been times when you could have had a cigarette or a second chocolate but you didn't. What probably happened is that neither you nor anyone else noticed this happening; or, if you did, you dismissed it as not good enough or just 'chance'. This is because we get into the bad habit of noticing problems and ignoring solutions, causing problems to get bigger and bigger so that any tiny improvements seem irrelevant. This is very discouraging for people with problems.

A solution focused conversation aims to discover even the smallest exception to the problem. Then the unique details of it are identified, such as what the person was thinking or doing that was different on those occasions, or when other people in their lives were being helpful. The purpose of this is to make those different circumstances much more visible and therefore memorable and accessible to use on the next occasion, with the aim of supporting the person in increasing the control they have over their problem and their life generally. The skill of the worker is in noticing the tiny beginnings of solutions and helping people 'literally talk themselves out of their troubles by encouraging them to describe their lives in new ways' (Miller 1997, p.6).

CASE EXAMPLE

Exceptions may be very small or not recognised or even discounted, especially where people have chronic difficulties. The only time Bridget had felt free from her depression was when she was on holiday abroad. This was not an experience she could repeat regularly but careful listening to the words she used to describe what being away was like revealed that the significance of being near water led to her being less depressed by dark thoughts. She could then identify smaller occasions when the depression was less, such as walking along a riverbank, and increase her coping strategy by taking up swimming, arranging trips to the seaside and buying a fish tank for her home.

Changing problem stories into solution stories

Talking is a powerful instrument, especially when workers are talking about lifelong conditions. A diagnosis of personality disorder or schizophrenia takes away a person's hope for meaningful recovery. In actual fact, 15 to 20 per cent of people have only one schizophrenic episode and, whilst many will need long-term support, over 60 per cent are stable in middle age, often without medication (for an overview, see Macdonald 2011, ch.8). Of course, many conditions are not only lifelong but deteriorating over time, but this does not mean that every day will be the same, that some days are not better than others.

When we describe something in negative terms, such as personality disorder, then we construct a negative image of the person as well as the problem. For example, Patrick was devastated to read the conclusions of his psychological report: 'Given his personality difficulties and the long-standing nature of his interpersonal problems, change is likely to be difficult to achieve...the prognosis is poor.' There is the danger here that people will begin to think of themselves as bad, or permanently damaged or incapable of being other than the negatives that they hear about themselves. Talking this way can also divide people into opposing sides when there are difficulties in relationships, viewing people as 'good' or 'bad' and reducing the opportunity for reconciliation and change. It also lends itself to blaming, where someone is seen as the problem rather than the product of, say, family dynamics. The tendency to see the world in binary categories usually means that someone is 'good' and therefore someone else is 'bad'.

These images and labels can limit people's potential for growth; for example, some men we have worked with tell us that they cannot 'do emotions' because of the way they were raised at the same time as being very emotionally upset by the consequences of this. The notion of an emotionally incompetent man is a powerful image of masculinity, often unhelpfully supported by partners, families and friends. We find that if we talk with them about a time when they coped with an emotional situation, or successfully negotiated a potentially difficult emotional conflict, and identify with them the skills and resources that they used, then the conversation shifts into one of optimism and achievement.

CASE EXAMPLE

Dave was violent to his partner and her family at home and on social outings. He found it difficult to think of a situation where he was not violent as he did not socialise outside the family circle and he worked mainly alone. Very occasionally he worked as part of a team and he was non-violent in that context. When asked how he did that, he replied that he treated his colleagues with respect. When asked how he 'did respect', he replied that he was polite and sociable. He was then asked if he could be polite and sociable towards his family, a task well within his capability in view of his behaviour when working in a team. At his second session, he recounted, with considerable pleasure, successful outings with his family that had included shopping, swimming and a trip to the park where he had been in complete control of his temper.

It is vital that the details of any exceptions are explored vigorously by asking what, when, where, how and who questions. Exploring for exceptions brings people's competences to their attention that may otherwise remain lost or hidden. People often tell us that they have no control over their temper, but can, when asked, give examples where their temper has been less of a problem or more under control. Within this context, questions related to what is different are relevant, focusing on what has been going well and how they did this so that they can do more of it. It also highlights to people that there have been successes (successes related to their hopes and best wishes and what's going well for them, and not successes which have been constructed and decided by people around them) and this is noticed.

Noticing progress and/or success is a very important skill in solution focused practice, especially where people with chronic difficulties seem to have plateaued. What has been noticed is discussed in a spirit of genuine curiosity: 'Tell me more about this' 'How did you do it?' 'Did anyone else notice this?' 'Was it hard or easy to do?' We do not praise people at this point or offer any suggestions as to how the person could do more of the exception. Instead, we would say something like, 'I'm impressed, are you?' The person may not at all be impressed and want more for themselves, so goals may need to be revisited. Where the person is pleased with the exception, we would say something like: 'Did you know this about yourself ?' or 'What does doing this tell you about you as a person?' This sort of conversation encourages the person to take responsibility for their own behaviour and to learn more about their personal qualities, skills and abilities.

CASE EXAMPLE

A very upset student came to see Steve. She was struggling to get her work in on time and was thinking about withdrawing from the course. She talked about having moved to the area to study following an acrimonious separation from her husband, bringing her three children with her but having few friends or family to support her. She described herself as lacking organisational skills and the focus necessary to complete the work.

Steve asked some gentle questions about how her children had all managed to get to school that day and what they liked for breakfast. She was able to describe her routine for getting the children up, getting washed, having clean clothes, making and eating breakfast, and organising with other parents to share getting the children to school. Steve asked how she had managed to do all that and they began to recognise the organisational skills, strength of character and commitment needed to achieve what she had with the children. They agreed that she would go and be less hard on herself and recognise that she had supermum skills that could translate into superstudent skills.

Steve left the university before she completed her degree, but he received a phone call two years later at his new place of work from her saying that she had just gained a first-class honours degree.

Such conversations increase the likelihood of hope and engagement and thus have potential for change. For example, when there are concerns about a parent's ability to meet a disabled child's needs it is much more productive to support changes and move things forward when the worker focuses on those times when the parent has met the child's needs, however fleetingly. In contrast, if the conversations consistently centre on the presence of unsafe behaviour, it is likely to promote 'problem talk' as well as make the parent feel like a failure, which could then move them into a position of thinking, 'What's the point?'

This is not to say that we should ignore unsafe or inappropriate behaviour as ultimately a vulnerable person's safety is of paramount importance; however, a useful question in this situation is, 'When things are going wrong, what do you do to put them right?' For example, if you were struggling with managing your time and the focus of the conversations with your manager was centred on your failure to get reports done on time or meet other deadlines, how would that make you feel? And how helpful would that be in supporting you in meeting deadlines in the future? Conversely, if the conversation focused on times when you have met, or come close to meeting deadlines, helping you discover what was different on those occasions, you are likely to feel more confident that you can do this again. Such a conversation would also help to bring your attention to a detailed plan of action that works best for you. Furthermore, discussions centred on what is/was different begin to construct a description of what life could be like and the differing experiences and possibilities.

CASE EXAMPLE

H. is a young woman with autism who has a lot of difficulties with changes. To move over from one task to another is very hard for her. As a teacher she finds it very stressful to change classes all the time. The restriction is: difficulties with transitions. We cannot make this go away. The problem here can be described as: being stressed when transitioning to different classes.

Together we explored ways to deal with this problem. We looked at what was helping in other moments that got her stressed. And it turned out that in other stressful situations, performing a little ritual helped her remain calm. A ritual she used at home to move on from one chore to the next was to drink a glass of water. She concluded herself that this was something she could do in school as well. She decided to drink half a glass of water after every class. This resulted in making the transition a lot easier for her. (Mattelin and Volckaert 2017)

Where someone can identify a deliberate exception and pinpoint specifically what and how they did it, the next question is obvious: 'Can you do more of it?' Lots of people have difficulty with answering 'how they did it' questions, however, saying things like, 'Well, I just did it,' or 'It just happened'; so, more questions are needed.

Prompt questions for when people are stuck include:

- Tell me about the times you are *not*...

- Tell me about the times you are *less*...

- Tell me about the times you can cope *despite* this feeling…

- When you feel like…and you don't, what do you do?

- How did you do that?

- Tell me about a time you refused to let [the problem] ruin your day.

- When was the last time you that you stopped [the problem] from spoiling your day?

- What will it be like when [the exception] is happening more?

- Who will notice when [the exception] is happening more?

- Who could help you do [the exception] more?

Where people have chronic or deteriorating conditions, the person can be invited to identify small exceptions:

- Tell me what is different on a better day.

- What does a good day look like?

- What helps you have a better day?

Some people persist in denying the existence of any exceptions, especially where they have got into the habit of viewing the problem as part of them, often through being told this is so by family or other professionals. This can be countered by expressing your amazement that they can maintain this state: 'What, you never get on with each other? Never? It must take a lot of commitment to make sure that you don't slip up and get on even a little. Sounds to me like a lot of hard work.' Then you can have a conversation about the person's ability to plan and work hard before moving the conversation lightly on to a more constructive tack with something like: 'Have you ever thought of having a short break from all this effort you are making every day?' As we mentioned earlier, humour is a useful tool, especially when someone doesn't want to back down from an entrenched position and lose face.

There are a few situations where the person genuinely cannot find an exception; for example, where someone has an extreme fear of needles. In these instances, success in a situation requiring the same resources can be explored, so we would ask questions such as, 'What is the bravest thing you have ever done?' Bravery is a transferable resource for tackling many problems. It is also useful to make enquiries of other people who are present in their lives as the following example shows.

CASE EXAMPLE

After her husband's sudden death from a heart attack, Bettina was off work for three months with severe depression, which was successfully treated with medication. Her family was very supportive during this period, visiting her frequently, taking her shopping and ringing to see how she was. As her return to work drew closer, Bettina began to experience acute anxiety. She extended her sick leave, becoming fearful of leaving the house unless accompanied by one of her daughters. Over the next few months, her condition worsened to such an extent that she could not face attending a return-to-work interview, instead handing in her notice. Two years on, she has become almost completely housebound, only venturing out when accompanied by one of her daughters and only to familiar places. Bettina desperately wants to attend her grandson's degree ceremony in two months' time but cannot face the lengthy car journey to an unfamiliar place, even if accompanied by her daughters.

Bettina is unable to think of a single exception to her anxiety so she is asked about the bravest thing she has ever done. She doesn't think she has ever done anything brave but her daughters are quick to point out several events, such as when she lifted a five-bar gate off her eldest daughter's leg when the gate fell on her and held it up until help arrived, and when she faced her fear of heights to rescue the family dog from a cliff fall. When asked what qualities these deeds took, Bettina shrugged off any notion that she had done anything special, saying, 'When it's life or death, you just do it.' As there was no life-or-death element to a university graduation ceremony, the worker asked for smaller examples of bravery. One daughter then told of Bettina going to the funeral of her cousin's wife. As the funeral party moved from the graveside, Bettina spontaneously left the side of her accompanying daughter and walked over to her cousin to offer sympathy. She then spoke with the priest and various mourners before looking to see where her daughter was.

This short, unaccompanied journey across the graveyard was a small but significant exception, which led to her realising that she had had control over her anxiety that day. And, therefore, she could 'do' it again.

PRACTICE ACTIVITY

Before you try this with the people with whom you work, try it on yourself. Next time you are struggling with something at home or at work, ask yourself the following questions:

- When have I coped when faced with a similar situation?

- What else was better?

- What was different on these occasions?

- What did I do that was different?

- How did I do this? (Name three things.)

- What else was happening?

- Who notices first when things are better?

- Who else?

- What do they notice at these times?

- What else?

- How would they know I was managing the situation in this preferred way?

- How can I do more of it?

- What else? (There is always more to discover.)

When having a conversation about 'what was different', you may find that it lends itself to looking at differences maybe two or three hours earlier. For example, if you have had a difficult morning at home before leaving for work, this is likely to put you in a different frame of mind than if you left home after an enjoyable calm breakfast. We have found that this is often the case when we track back to look at the differences with young children when their behaviour has been more appropriate at school than on previous occasions. There will often be some reference to being up on time, sitting down for breakfast, having a nice conversation, having fun, being relaxed, people talking in a nice way.

When we are training practitioners in this way of working, we are often asked to do a live demonstration. We ask for a volunteer with a small problem and almost invariably the small problem turns out to be one of time poverty in the morning, leading to raised voices, arguments and upset.

Exception finding when people have little or no language

As you will have seen, solution focused work is heavily premised on the use of language. When someone has limited language skills, this may at first appear to undermine the whole approach; for example, when someone is either physically or intellectually disabled and struggles to talk. Lloyd *et al.* (2016) describe ways in which solution focused techniques can be adapted to provide creative and useful practice in these instances, making interventions that are better described as being 'informed by solution-oriented thinking' (p.65). They suggest making behavioural observations to see how the person already successfully adapts and responds to their needs, using behavioural records to chart what they did and what was happening around the person at times when the problem was less of a problem. This can include noting the specific setting, the interactional style, what happened in the run-up to the exception and what happened following this. The observer can retain a strengths focus by asking the question, 'What helps this person be so good?' (p.65).

Bliss (2012) provides the example of a woman resident in a home for people with autism spectrum disorder whose behaviours included screaming, self-injuring, rocking and playing with bodily fluids. As she did not speak, a solution focused approach was taken with the caring staff, where they were invited to discuss their preferred future for her and those times when her behaviour had been less of a problem (exceptions) and when she had responded positively to particular interventions. From these conversations a clearer picture of which interactions were more helpful for her emerged, enabling the staff to do more of these.

Exception finding when everyone is being negative

Where someone has 'become the problem', people in their lives have been living with failure and criticism too and may well have become very negative. They can become so familiar with, and ground down by, the problem that they may find it difficult to recognise exceptions; or they dismiss them as insignificant now that the problem has become so big. In these situations it helps first of all to notice what people are doing right, and acknowledge this. This could relate to something specific, such as the person being polite (however briefly), in which case you could say something like, 'Gosh, how nice to meet someone who knows about good manners. [Addressing the family] Manners are obviously important in your family.' Or it could be something as basic as noticing that they are still looking for a solution: 'Despite all that this problem has put you through, you're still here for your son. This says a lot about your determination and caring when faced with his drug abuse.' Should the family still find it difficult to acknowledge any exceptions, you can shift the emphasis by changing how the negative information is collected.

CASE EXAMPLE

Evelyn is 67 years old and has had Parkinson's disease for several years. She has been admitted to hospital with swallowing and communication difficulties. She is unable to identify any times when her situation is improved but the speech therapist persists in exception finding:

> Therapist: When do you feel your communication is working a bit better?
>
> Evelyn: I don't get much opportunity to talk. I've never been good at it... It's difficult, I'm stuck in a chair.
>
> Therapist: I'm sorry to hear things are so difficult for you. How have you managed to cope in such difficult circumstances?
>
> Evelyn: I don't know... I don't like people treating me like a baby. At the Day Centre they would compliment me on filling in one or two words in a crossword puzzle...
>
> Therapist: What would be the best way to show them you're not a baby?
>
> Evelyn: They could wait until I've completed the crossword. If people talk over my head, I say 'Meow!'

(Adapted from Burns 2016, pp.30–31)

Externalising problems

Workers can't always get resources for people with problems and difficulties unless they fit specific categories or have been diagnosed with an illness or disability. However useful, this can have a negative effect in that the category or diagnosis may become a label that describes the whole person; for example, he's autistic, she's anorexic. Some people are oppressed by the labels they have grown up with; for example, Jessica hoped to become a secretary but, unable to see past her mild learning difficulties, her social worker suggested that she stop dreaming and get a job in a supermarket. Other people learn to collude with the label; for example, 'I'm no good at making friends because I've got Asperger's' or 'I struggle to maintain relationships because of my anxious-ambivalent attachment style.'

Of course, people are not simply anorexics, or drug addicts, or diabetics, or whatever the label; they are people who just happen to have a problem. To help us to remain focused on the individual in the face of labelling, we use a narrative therapy technique called *externalisation* (White and Epston 1990). This is a technique whereby the person is separated from the problem through a problem-naming process, which enables people to see that problems are not internal to them, nor are their identities shaped by, or reflections of, the problems they are experiencing. This is a powerful and empowering alternative way of talking about problems, one with which people rapidly engage.

CASE EXAMPLE

Sophia suffered from extreme eczema, which became much worse after she was teased about it at school. It was so bad at night that she was unable to sleep for more than an hour or so. Her parents were having to stay awake to secure her hands so she couldn't do further damage to her flesh. Her medications were nearing toxic levels so her doctor referred her to the narrative therapist, David Epston, to see if Sophia could be helped to prevent eczema from controlling her consciousness.

At his first meeting with the family, David noticed that Sophia was dealing with the problem in front of his eyes. She said she had a fair bit of itchiness on her arms so David remarked that as she was not sitting on her hands, she must be using her mind to stop herself from itching. This was the beginning of a separation of Sophia from her problem, which she then began talking about as The Itch and how she could get angry at The Itch rather than getting angry with her skin.

Over several sessions, Sophia and David explored how The Itch operated on her, what tactics it used to make her life miserable and what qualities and abilities she used to defeat it. Whilst it is easier to distract oneself from scratching during the day, it is much more difficult at night. However, Sophia's ability to gain some control over The Itch resulted in her being able to get a full night's sleep.

> (Adapted from Freeman, Epston and Lobovits 1997; for a full account of the externalising conversation between David and Sophia, see pp.265–277. This text also contains an account of externalising in the case of 'Ben', whose nausea and vomiting was so severe that he had not been able to take food orally for six months; see pp.20–33.)

Opportunities are provided to the person to 'name' the problem in such a way that it is relevant and meaningful to them. Metaphors that fit with the person's speech patterns are then introduced into the conversation, so you may talk about fighting the problem with one person whereas with another you would be talking about taking control. Then details are collected about how the person has achieved this previously – exception finding. Such conversations provide alternative stories, ones about how the person has confronted the problem successfully in the past. Successful strategies give hope and acknowledgement that there have been periods, however small, of things going well.

Communicating about 'problems' can be difficult. One of the first hurdles is actually acknowledging and openly discussing what is wrong. Naming the problem can provide a safe vocabulary for family members to feel able to discuss their worries and begin to find ways of managing their difficulties. This is especially important where a problem is beginning to seem intractable; a situation whereby blame is beginning to entrench feelings and the ability to see change. Externalising takes blame out of the picture as it changes everyone's relationship with the problem. Once the problem has been named and understood, everyone can gang up on the problem rather than the person. It can also take the stigma out of the situation.

CASE EXAMPLE

Kate Swaffer externalises her early onset dementia:

> if you think of dementia as we do in my house, and that 'it' is the third person in the threesome, it could be seen

as us both living with 'it'. And we call this troublesome threesome the Three Stooges, and have even named 'it', Larry!' (2016, p.202)

This paves the way for externalising her 'carer':

In 2012 I nicknamed my husband BUB, or Back-Up Brain, and we find this terminology far easier to live with than carer or even care partner... My husband says he cared for me long before I had dementia, and objects to this title or label. He is my best friend and husband, and sometimes he supports me. Sometimes I support him. That is what friends and couples do. Hence the term BUB. He is my best friend and husband, and to start calling him my 'carer' simply denigrates us both. (2016, p.240)

Mapping the problem

An externalising conversation begins with a description of the problem (identifying an appropriate name for the problem); consideration of the effects of the problem on the person; an evaluation of these effects; and then, a justification of the evaluation. It is important that the person names the behaviour as it is the naming that makes the situation unique to them and supports a description from how they see the problem: 'If you were to give this problem we are talking about a name, what would you call it?' When considering the effects, this exploration encourages the person to see the problem as separate from them and their identity: 'At times when the [named] problem is more in control of what happens, how has it affected different areas/relationships in your life?'

The next step is to provide an opportunity for the person to evaluate the effects that they have been describing. These questions provide a space for them to reflect on whether these effects are something that they are happy about or not, and as such leads on to justification questions, which begin to get a richer description of what is important to them. So, for example, a conversation with someone who is misusing substances could include these questions:

- Is cannabis for or against you?

- How did cannabis con you into thinking that you need it in your life?

- What influence does cannabis have on your life, on those close to you, on your relationships?

- Given a choice between life with cannabis or life free of cannabis, which do you choose?

- What prevented you from resisting cannabis? How did cannabis use these things to move into your life?

- How much of your life will cannabis be satisfied with, or does it want the lot?

- Does it suit you to be dominated by cannabis?

- Tell me about a time when you didn't fall for the lies cannabis has been telling you.

- Tell me about times when you made cannabis wait.

- What does it say about you as a person when you refuse to cooperate with cannabis's invitations?

- In the times when you have felt in control of cannabis, what are the things that helped you have that control?

- Tell me about a time when cannabis didn't stop you being in touch with your hopes and dreams.

PRACTICE ACTIVITY

Think of a mildly compulsive behaviour or habit you have, such as shopping, smoking, indulging in 'wine o'clock', rechecking that you have locked the door when you go out, as you ask yourself the questions listed above.

CASE EXAMPLE

Jane binges on diets almost as often as she binges on food. She is overweight and unhappy. She externalises her binge eating as *The Comfort Monster* because binge eating has advantages for her (stopping at home with a box set and a large tub of ice cream is comforting because it means she doesn't have to go out and feel horribly self-conscious on the dance floor) and disadvantages (it puts weight on her, makes her feel bad about herself and stops her going out with friends). She is overwhelmed by the problem to the extent that she can't set a goal for herself because she is sure that she will fail. The worker suggests they interview The Comfort Monster to get to know better how it operates on her and model how Jane could stand up to it:

Worker [as Jane]: I think I'll make myself a salad for supper tonight.

Jane [as The Comfort Monster]: Ho, ho, ho. Here we go again. Starting another diet, are we?

Worker [as Jane]: So what if I am?

Jane [as The Comfort Monster]: You know what will happen. It won't fill you up, you'll be starving later. But it's all right. I'll be there for you, we can have some crisps later. And there's that tub of chocolate ice cream. We can all settle down and watch television and you won't need to hold a cushion in front of your stomach because it'll just be you and me.

Worker [as Jane]: I'm making a lettuce and egg salad so there will be enough protein to keep me feeling full. I won't be hungry.

Jane [as The Comfort Monster]: Oooh, egg salad. Make sure you don't forget to smother it with lots of lovely mayonnaise. And some crusty bread and butter would be nice, too. We're going to have a great evening.

Worker [as Jane]: No, that would make me feel bloated. And, anyway, I'm going out tonight with my mates so I don't have time for a big meal.

Jane [as The Comfort Monster]: You know you won't enjoy it. As soon as you start trying on different outfits, you'll get all upset that nothing fits and they make you look fat. Better stay in with me. I like the way you look.

Worker [as Jane]: It's all your fault they don't fit. I'm sick of you making me fat. There, I've said it – fat, fat, fat.

Jane [as The Comfort Monster]: Fat – and ugly and useless. If you go out, they'll all be talking about you behind your back. I'm your true friend. Come on, let's have our evening in. I tell you what, we could have a bottle of wine as well. And you can put your slippers on and that comfy dressing gown and we will be sooo comfy.

Worker [as Jane]: I've had enough of you bossing me about and making me feel bad about myself.

Jane [as The Comfort Monster]: And so you should feel bad about yourself. What's good about you anyway? You're a total failure. If it wasn't for me, you wouldn't have anyone.

PRACTICE ACTIVITY

Continue this dialogue for at least three more exchanges between the worker [you as Jane] and Jane [as The Comfort Monster].

(For examples of externalising conversations with anorexia, see Jacob 2001, pp.66–68.)

Externalising with people who just can't think of a name for their problem

Most people find it easy to name their problem, but some with a learning difficulty can find it puzzling. Ways of helping people in these situations include drawing or modelling the problem, which then makes the problem more visual and therefore easier for the person to take a stand against. Where people really struggle to think of a name, we sometimes suggest names that other people have used and ask if one of the names fits for the person. When they borrow a name for their problem, we remind them that they can change it at any time. Or you can ask the person what animal or film/TV character the problem is most like. One young man found it much easier to tolerate the demands of his disabled brother once he had identified him as a hippogriff and himself as Harry Potter. As any Harry Potter fan knows, hippogriffs are wonderfully talented animals but require very careful and sensitive handling. The next step was to ask the young man what hippogriff-handling skills he already has, and what skills he needs to develop.

For people with learning difficulties, we have used an extension of the Mr. Men characters. These have the advantage of being simple to draw (which is helpful for us as well, as we are not talented in this area), needing no more than a circle for the body and line drawings for arms and legs, and a defining characteristic. The defining characteristic is the problem; for example, you may help a person design a *Miss Can't Be*

Bothered or a *Mr Just Do It*. Then you can ask the person for exceptions: 'Tell me about a time when *Miss Can't Be Bothered* tried to get you to miss your medication, but you didn't,' followed by questions about how the person did it. This can be made visual for the person by designing an opposite Mr. Man figure; for example, *Miss Can't Be Bothered* might be countered by *Miss Thoughtful*. *Mr Just Do It* could be countered with a *Mr Think First*. Soon you are well towards a story in which *Miss Can't Be Bothered* or *Mr Just Do It* gets their comeuppance (for a more fully worked example, see Milner 2008b, pp.47–48).

Some people who are violent or anti-social can struggle to externalise their problem behaviours, often preferring to see the problem as who they are. This may be because of the way they have been dealt with by their family and previous professionals, supported by common social and psychological explanations of poor behaviour ('I'm just a psycho!'), or because they gain some credibility from the label ('He is a psycho – give him respect!'). In these situations, it is possible to interview the problem; for example, 'What does "psycho" get you to do that makes life better for you?' or 'When does "psycho" appear?', What does "psycho" like and what makes it stronger?' or 'What does "psycho" dislike?' or 'What problems does "psycho" cause for you?' which explore all the effects that 'psycho' has in their life. This approach recognises that problems are complex and can have benefits as well as negatives, which will resonate with the person's lived experience and lend credibility to the conversation.

Similarly, some people have become so used to being described as a problem that they have become quite hopeless. For example, although tackling obesity is a clear health priority, few existing interventions appear to work (Licence 2005), although disapproval of being fat remains. Obesity is also a problem that is embarrassing, and it can be easier for fat people if 'fatness' is interviewed, rather than themselves.

Exception finding in safeguarding

By the nature of your organisation, every person with whom you work is a vulnerable adult. Your role in ensuring they live in safety, free from abuse and neglect is spelled out in the government publication *Statement of Government Policy on Adult Safeguarding* (DoH 2011) and the Care Act 2014. Engaging people in a conversation about how best to respond to their safeguarding situation in a way that enhances involvement, choice and control as well as improving quality of life, well-being and safety – within the framework of the Mental Capacity Act (2005) – is exactly what solution focused practice is all about.

Being person-centred and outcome focused can be problematic for some workers; just how do they allow people to make choices about their care and treatment, even when those decisions may seem to others to be unwise (being person-centred) at the same time as delivering safety outcomes? Here the solution focused Signs of Safety approach pioneered in child protection work (Turnell and Edwards 1999; Turnell and Essex 2006; see www.signsofsafety.com) ensures that the safety goals of all concerned people are included. A Signs of Safety assessment documents both concerns and safety alongside canvassing the goals and perspectives of both professionals and family members. The focus is on developing and increasing the level of safety to the point that all the concerns are answered with measurable outcomes. At the heart of this approach is exception finding.

As we mentioned earlier, no problem happens all the time but where a person's safety is in doubt, workers' responsibility to ensure that no further harm occurs tends to focus them on what has gone wrong. Thus safeguarding work can become totally dominated by the abuse that happened and the risk of it happening again. This is to ignore the fact that abusive behaviour doesn't happen all the time. It is in developing these exceptions that safety can be found. Exceptions are the first signs of safety so it is important to discover these early on and expand them until there is sufficient safety that is tangible and measurable.

It is important to ask questions such as, 'Tell me about a time when you felt your temper rising when [person's name] was being particularly difficult to feed and you felt like leaving them hungry, but you didn't? What were you doing differently at that time? Can you do more of it?' or 'Tell me about a time when your caring is really good. What do other people notice you doing when they see you doing really good care? How can you do more of this?' Exceptions do not guarantee safety but they do form a constructive starting point for developing a safety plan. They also engage people who might otherwise be unwilling to talk about the situation if your focus is entirely on what they have done or are doing wrong.

It is especially important to focus on exceptions at case conferences and reviews, otherwise you will find yourself discussing risk for

95 per cent of the meeting and only 5 per cent of your time will be spent on safety planning. Furthermore, the identification of what works for families, homes and hospitals to make them safer and healthier places will be more meaningful to everyone and thus increase the likelihood of safer behaviour being sustained in the future. Where there are no exceptions, there is increased danger and people will need to be removed from their situations.

CASE EXAMPLE

Re-read the example of Lena and Mark in Chapter 1 (see p.33). Nursing staff were so concerned about Lena's safety that they wanted her to be discharged to a care home where she would be safe from (probable) physical assaults by Mark. Mark was defensive when questioned about his mother's bruises, saying she fell over a lot. He visited his mother regularly in hospital, bringing her a huge box of chocolates, which she proudly showed other patients, saying what a loving son she had. Staff were of the opinion that this was a sign of his guilt. Lena insisted on returning to her home with Mark – making a person-centred decision that seemed to others to be unwise. To ensure a good safety outcome, the worker met with Lena and Mark at home and began developing a safety plan.

The worker commented that they obviously had a lot of love for each other, choosing to live together despite all the difficulties they were experiencing, acknowledging that Mark had debts, no job, no home of his own and a lot of care responsibility for one so young, and Lena's losses of her husband and health. The worker wondered how they coped with all these pressures and what qualities they might have that could have been forgotten under all the current pressures. She then focused her conversation on times when Mark's care was good. And there were plenty of times when Lena found his care very good, indeed. Mark was able to explain how he did good care, and talk freely about times when his care fell far short of good – mostly when he was tired and depressed about his own situation.

PRACTICE ACTIVITY

Make a list of your, Lena's and Mark's concerns and needs. What sort of help do you think is needed to meet these needs and what measurable outcomes would be required to remove your concerns?

Incidents of abuse of older people in care homes in the interests of staff convenience (tying people to chairs, putting people to bed early) or the financial abuse of older people in their own homes is often highlighted in the press, but a vulnerable person's well-being can be compromised in much more subtle ways. These are much harder to detect and, where there is emotional abuse, often more damaging than physical abuse. For example, disrespecting people with dementia through nasty teasing will result in those people's well-being and cognitive capacity declining rapidly. Searching for evidence of such abuse is difficult; it is far easier to look for the key sign of safety – well-being: is this person as physically well as possible, are they well nourished, are they smiling, are they eating? And, if not, what could be happening differently to improve matters?

And, of course, there is always institutional abuse, so we leave you with a challenging practice activity.

PRACTICE ACTIVITY

Recalling the case of Bill and Peggy described in Chapter 2 (see p.59), following Bill having another heart attack, the couple are accommodated in a care home. Bill asks for them to be allowed to go home with domiciliary help but is told that they would need so much help that it would cost more than staying in the home and the social care budget won't cover it:

- What can you do to assist Bill and Peggy in making choices about their care and treatment?

Key points

- The basic premise of solution focused practice is that there are always exceptions to problems (although this can be to varying degrees and take different forms). The challenge for the worker is to listen actively for those times when exceptions have occurred, but may have been missed or not considered significant by the person; or to ask the questions and make the necessary inquiry to enable the person to have the opportunity to think and identify times when the problem hasn't happened or happened less. This conversation to identify specifically what was different is then strengthened by amplifying the details that focus on the where, when, what, how and who.

- Having these conversations is for the purpose of making these successes, and specifically what the person did to make them happen, more visible so that they can build upon them and apply them within their daily routines.

- Locating exceptions can be an uplifting and powerful experience for people, particularly when they believe or have been told that they are 'failures'. Considering people's successes is also the best confirmation to them that there have been times when things have gone well.

Chapter Five

Discovering People's Strengths

Effective work with people is helped by making their strengths and abilities more evident to them and to others who are important in their lives. Identifying these resources provides material for finding each person's unique solutions to their problems and also develops their resilience. This chapter begins with a brief discussion of the nature and characteristics of resilience and then describes different ways of discovering people's skills, aptitudes and abilities. It also outlines how behaviours that on the surface appear to be deficits can be converted into strengths. As well as case examples, there are also activities to enable readers to (re)discover their own skills and resources.

Strengths and resilience

In concentrating on searching for solutions, we are sometimes accused of ignoring problems at our peril. We are told that our work is superficial, that problems have to be explored at length and in depth or that they will be papered over, only to re-emerge later. After all, ignoring problems doesn't make them go away. Unlike plumbing problems, however, people's problems don't necessarily have any link whatsoever with the solutions they devise. Even where there is a direct link between a problem and a solution, such as obesity and diabetes, plans for eating more healthily will vary significantly from person to person.

When our toilet breaks, we want an expert plumber to come in and fix it. Some people view professional helpers like this and expect a metaphorical toolkit to appear and mend their pain or problem; however, we consider that people have their own ideas how to fix themselves and have their preferred solutions to their problems, with strengths, skills and abilities to develop those solutions. In short, everyone is an expert in their problems and in their solutions, although they may not yet recognise it. A central part of our work concentrates on helping people to discover these resources.

PRACTICE ACTIVITY

Originally a bricklayer, 48-year-old Antonin has been receiving kidney dialysis at a specialist hospital unit some ten miles from his home. He has been off work for three years. Today, he is having a pre-operation assessment prior to receiving a kidney transplant. Whilst the physical tests are being administered, the nurse assesses Antonin's physical and mental strengths that may increase his resilience to the possible effects of major surgery:

- Prepare a list of possible questions you might ask Antonin.

Following the Winterbourne View scandal of systematic abuse of people with learning disabilities, the Skills for Care & Skills for Health (2014) produced guidance on reducing the need for restrictive practices. One of the key principles was recognising that 'understanding people's behaviour allows their unique needs, aspirations, experiences and *strengths* to be recognised and their quality of life to be enhanced' (p.1, our emphasis). People with intellectual disabilities are often viewed as deficit-saturated where strengths and capabilities are presumed to be lacking. Similarly, assessments of older people are often focused on deficits yet despite functional deficits, 'older people demonstrate remarkable resiliency. They often possess an underutilized or untapped capacity for growth and change even in the context of difficult life challenges' (Nelson-Becker *et al.* 2013, p.165). Our approach supports the guidance in providing a presumption that everyone has strengths and we need to look for them to support people effectively; maintaining or expanding capacity is always the goal.

To use a medical analogy, if we think of problems like tumours, there are two ways of tackling them. We can be problem focused and get them out, expose them through surgery, dissect them in order to discover their pathology, stitch up the holes, and wait for the scars to fade. Or we can boost people's immune systems so that tumours are dissipated. Solution focused approaches take the latter view and attempt to boost people's resilience so that they can take the lead in reaching a problem-free future. Some people cope with setbacks very well, whether they are small ones, such as failing an essay, or big ones, such as living with a progressive condition such as motor neurone disease. Their resilience helps them pick themselves up and get on with life.

PRACTICE ACTIVITY

Lulé *et al.* (2009) studied patients who had locked-in syndrome (LIS), that is, they were awake and conscious but almost entirely without the ability to move or verbally communicate. They found that despite their impairments and the expectations of those around them, the patients maintained they had a good quality of life when questioned in ways that they were able to respond to using assistive technology. Their quality of life and level of depression were unrelated to their physical functioning and were similar to those of healthy individuals in their age range:

- What do you think made these patients so resilient to their severe physical limitations?

CASE EXAMPLE

For a moving example of resilience in someone who experienced locked-in syndrome, see Marsh and Hudson 2014.

Other people don't cope at all well; they get stuck, see life as very unfair, and sometimes become depressed or begin self-harming. The difference between these two groups of people is not the severity of their problems; it is the ability to get a good outcome in the face of adversity. We consider it important to help people become more resilient because they need to be able to cope with what life throws at them, adapt to testing situations, take appropriate responsibility and continue to develop.

We avoid spending too much time on problems, because this is a negative approach that has the effect of making us think negatively about the person. Thinking negatively about the person does not help us discover the strengths and resources that can be developed into their personal resilience. People thinking negatively about themselves (those who are pessimistic), get depressed more often and achieve less in life, and their physical health is worse (Selekman 2007). Assuming that the opposite of negative can only be positive, however, is insulting to people facing life-threatening situations and a range of emotions.

CASE EXAMPLE

On being diagnosed with breast cancer, Judith found herself on the receiving end of exhortations to 'be positive' and 'reassured' with comments such as 'you'll be okay, my auntie had what you've got and she's fine now'. Such comments vastly oversimplify the complexities of people's situations; after all, there are many different sorts of breast cancer with very differing likely outcomes and emotional responses to treatment options fluctuate widely. Judith decided that she had no intention whatsoever of 'staying positive'. Instead, she decided to respond to her situation with stubbornness and grumpiness, characteristics that sat easily with her. (Milner "Don't tell me how I should feel about my breast cancer" 2008a)

We will explain how we go about building resilience, but first, we spend a little time looking at the characteristics of resilience:

1. *Maintaining good relationships with close family members, friends and others* is a key element of resilience. Helping others and being open to being helped are activities that strengthen resilience, and taking an active part in faith, social, civic or other groups enhances a sense of worth. As Howe says, 'many of life's major resiliences are acquired in the context of close relationships, particularly parent–person and peer relationships' (2008, p.107), so working to strengthen these ties is an important investment for future emotional health.

2. *Avoiding seeing crises or stressful events as unbearable problems.* Stressful events happen, this is simply life in action, and we can have little control over these; however, we can have some control over how we respond to, and understand, events. When faced with such situations, we can ensure that we keep an eye to a future when the problem will be less (for example, grief at a loss does get less pronounced with time) and make sure that we are aware of our successes, no matter how small, in dealing with the problem. People who can stay involved rather than withdrawing are more likely to be

able to keep trying to influence events rather than give up. They also learn that stress is a challenge to be faced rather than bemoaning their fate. This involves seeing themselves accurately so that they can distinguish between problems that are their own fault, taking responsibility to try to correct the behaviour, and still feeling worthwhile when problems are not their fault (Selekman 2007).

3. *Accepting that some circumstances cannot be changed.* Life is not always fair and there are some situations which cannot be altered. Rather than generating frustration and loss of motivation by continuing to expend energy in a fruitless task, it is better to accept that it is time to focus on something that you can change.

4. *Developing realistic goals and moving towards them.* Having ambitions, goals, a desire for achievement and motivation helps people believe that things will be better in the future. This is why goal setting is so important in solution focused work, and why goals do not need to be limited to an immediate problem but can be much broader. It is important to generate motivation to reach the goals and to recognise (and celebrate) your progress in getting there. The actions do not need to be big – small moves towards the goal are still in the right direction.

5. *Taking decisive actions in adverse situations.* Rather than 'freezing', being overwhelmed by or ignoring problem situations, make sure that you engage with them and take whatever action is required to begin to deal with them.

6. *Looking for opportunities for self-discovery after a struggle with loss.* When dealing with adversity, people can often find strengths that they did not know they had. Being open to recognising this is helpful in enabling people to take new directions in their lives and find new ways of coping with difficult situations and events.

7. *Developing self-confidence.* Learning to recognise and trust your skills and competences in solving problems and coping with adversity is an important part of improving your resilience.

There are often influences on us (parental, familial, social) that can damage or limit our self-confidence, and this in turn can make us more prone to defeat and dismay. Confidence develops from previous successes that remind people of how they have overcome adversity in the past, which is why one question we ask a great deal is, 'Can you tell me how you handled problems before?' or 'What is the hardest thing you have ever done?' And, of course, 'How did you do it?' and 'Can you do it again?'

8. *Keeping a long-term perspective and considering the stressful event in a broader context.* When difficult events happen, they can often feel overwhelming and it can be hard to see an end to them. It is helpful to use techniques to locate the event within a broader view, thus avoiding the tendency to totalise and catastrophise the event and also seeing that change can happen.

9. *Maintaining a hopeful outlook, expecting good things and visualising what is wished.* Being cheerful and positive (often with a sense of humour) are beneficial attributes, and having a clear vision and purpose provides drive and energy.

10. *Taking care of one's mind and body, exercising regularly, paying attention to one's own needs and feelings.* It can be easy to neglect ourselves both emotionally and physically, and this can impact on how we feel. Women can be pressured into focusing on other people to the exclusion of their own needs, and men can be encouraged to behave in self-destructive ways (for example, heavy drinking) through expectations of masculinity. These pressures can be difficult to resist but we know that self-care is something that has a broad impact on how we function and feel, and being kind to ourselves can strengthen our ability to develop resilience (see also Haines 2015 [trauma]; Lahad, Shacham and Ayalon 2012 [PTSD]; MacKinlay and Trevitt 2012 [dementia]; Tizard and Clarke 2000; Timmins forthcoming [autism]).

PRACTICE ACTIVITY

How resilient are you as a worker? Look at the list of resilience skills below and then answer the questions:

1. Having a sense of humour. Reivich and Shatte (2003) say that this is an important skill but that it can't be learned; however, other resilience skills are all learnable.

2. Emotional awareness – the ability to identify what you are feeling and, when necessary, the ability to control your feelings. In solution focused terms, this would be described as not being able to help how you feel, but being responsible for how you behave when you have these feelings.

3. Impulse control – the ability to tolerate ambiguity so that you don't rush to make decisions, but rather that you look at things thoughtfully.

4. Optimism that is wedded to reality in that you don't simply look on the 'bright side' all the time. Instead, an optimistic explanatory style helps you think about an adverse experience in a constructive way; namely, it's a temporary setback.

5. Possess the ability to look at problems from many perspectives.

6. The ability to read and understand emotions is a social competence that provides social support. Resilient adults don't necessarily go it alone; they know when to ask for help and where to go for that help.

7. Self-efficacy. Confidence in your own ability to solve problems, knowing your strengths and weaknesses, and relying on the former to cope. This is a skills-based notion of coping that is different from self-esteem, which is to do with judgements about self-worth.

8. Reaching out and being prepared to take appropriate risk is also a characteristic of resilience. This means having a willingness to try things and considering failure as a part of life.

You don't need all of these skills to be resilient, so:

- Select one skill from this list that you are strong on.

- Think how you can use it more.

- What will you be doing differently when you are using this skill more?

- What will other people notice differently about you?

Conversations about strengths

People who deal well with difficult situations analyse a problem, decide on a solution and plan how to carry out this solution, revising the plan when necessary. Thus, says Howe (2008), they use their intellectual, emotional and practical strengths. So they need to become aware of the resources they already possess that can be used in the solution, and which resources need a little more development.

CASE EXAMPLE

I went blind suddenly when I was 75. I can remember it clearly – it was on the day of the royal wedding. I thought the world had finished for me. I didn't think I could be any use to anyone anymore. I had always been so active. I used to go dancing two or three times a week. When you lose your sight, you feel nobody is interested in you. You feel your life is finished. *But I'm the sort of person that likes a challenge. If anyone says I can't do this or I can't do that, I like to have a go.* Getting a guide dog is the best thing that happened to me. It gave me back my independence. Now nearly 90, I still live on my own. I have a home help two hours a week, I still go to a nearby old people's home for my lunch four days a week, and go out every day with my guide dog. (Lewycka 2002, p.34, our emphasis)

We therefore have an intense interest in people's competences away from the problem, and how these can be increased. Talking about what's going well in a person's life and the strengths and resources used in that also engages the person in a collaborative relationship with you; people enjoy talking about their successes, and don't always get much opportunity to do so.

People with problems do not expect to be valued or have their skills and abilities explored, so a conversation about these provides a balance for those people who are overwhelmed by failure. A strengths conversation consists of: first, the discovery of the person's skills, qualities and resources; second, that these are acknowledged and validated via carefully constructed compliments. It is rare that the solution focused worker offers a direct compliment, such as 'well done', 'that's fantastic' and so on. These sorts of compliments tend to lead on to 'keep it up', thus missing out an important part of the conversation about how the person achieved the success and what resources were most useful. These aspects are essential if the person is to become more aware of the qualities they can bring to bear on their problems. Direct compliments also have the disadvantage of making the person dependent on your praise, whereas what you are aiming for is to encourage them to compliment themselves, as they recognise their own strengths and potential. And, of course, people who are poor at receiving criticism are usually poor at accepting compliments too, tending to shrug them off: 'He's just being nice to me,' rather than being able to recognise successful actions or parts of themselves.

Indirect compliments, however, can be used until people are able to compliment themselves. Solution focused compliments are not the same as positive reinforcement, ego strengthening, praise or positive thinking. They are simply a means of validating the resources that people have discovered about themselves and put to good use. A commonly used indirect compliment is to repeat what resources the person has identified in response to the question, 'How did you do that?' and then say, 'Did you know that about yourself?' So, an indirect compliment fits into a strengths conversation something like this:

- 'You managed to meet your work deadlines all last week. Gosh! How did you do that?'

- 'You tell me that you just did it but there must be more to it than that. What made you stick at it? Could it have been concentration? Determination? Something else?'

- 'Aha, you kept yourself away from distractions. That's new for you, isn't it?'

- 'Did you know that when you keep yourself free from distractions, you can concentrate and get a load of work done?'

- 'Well, you do now! That says a lot about you as a person. Can you use this keeping yourself free from distractions skill in other parts of your problem?'

There are many varieties of strengths conversations, but before we describe some of them, first we invite you to have a strengths conversation with yourself by undertaking the exercises below.

PRACTICE ACTIVITY

1. Sparkling moments.

   This is an exercise developed by BRIEF (www.brief.org.uk), which, in turn, is based on ideas from narrative therapy (http://dulwichcentre. com.au)

   - Think of a time when you were at your best, when you felt 'sparkling'. Describe it briefly.

   - What was it in particular about that moment which caused it to stand out?

   - What are you most pleased to remember about yourself at that moment?

   - What else were you pleased to notice? What else? What else?

   - If these qualities were to play an even bigger part in your life, who would be the first to notice?

   - What would they see?

   - What difference would that make?

2. Ever appreciating circles (from Hackett 2005, p.84).

   Purpose:

   - to allow you to notice the minutiae of competencies in your daily situations

   - to help you learn to look at the world with an appreciative eye rather than focusing on deficits.

Look for things people do that you appreciate, particularly those hidden right in front of you. When you see them, acknowledge them verbally or non-verbally. Then pay attention to any evidence of an appreciative circle rippling back to you.

Questions:

- What do you notice at home that you appreciate?

- What do you notice about your colleagues and friends that you appreciate?

- Without people saying anything, in what ways do they make your day?

- What effect does it have on you?

- When you tell them what you appreciate about them, what difference do you notice about them physically, verbally?

- When you notice an appreciative circle rippling back to you, what difference does it make to you?

How to get a strengths conversation going

The simplest way to begin the conversation is to show curiosity about strengths by making a deliberate shift from problem talk. You could say something like, 'You've told me a lot about your problem, but if we are going to find out how to fix it, I need to know what's going well for you right now. Then we can use what's going well to fix all this stuff that's not going so well.' Or, more simply, you could ask the person to tell you what the good things about them are. Very often, people will respond to this question with puzzlement, saying they don't know, or that there isn't anything good about them. Some follow-up questions to help them find the good things include:

- What would your friends say are the good things about you?

- What would your mum/dad/partner/children say are the good things about you?

- What would your best friend say?

- If your dog/cat/gerbil could talk, what would they say are the good things about you?

- What are you good at?

- What is the hardest thing you have ever done?

- What else?

- What else?

All these questions are followed up with an expression of curiosity about how the person achieved their successes, identifying the skills, personal qualities and resources they used, however small and seemingly insignificant. It is important to take your time over this conversation and be thorough, as people find it a little strange at first. Until they have developed the ability to compliment themselves, it is your task to ferret out their strengths. This can require persistence, as the following extract in the case example demonstrates.

CASE EXAMPLE

Richard is 24 years old and has Down's syndrome. His mother's health was precarious so there were major concerns about how Richard might deal with losing his mother. As Richard communicates in ways that are not always understood by others, his worker set up a special working folder containing lists, charts, stories, letters and poetry. The worker learned that Richard had experienced many changes in his life so she talked with him about how 'big' each was in his life and how he got used to them.

Richard said he thought he managed the big changes because he was competent – being strong, like having 'inside muscles' and 'outside muscles' – and by having people on his side when he needed them. As he had a very big change coming up – his mother was his main carer – his 'inside muscles' will provide the strength for him to deal with the change, and its accompanying grief. (Brown and Brown 2003, p.199; for the full case study, see pp.197–204).

The inclusion of others in identifying, recognising and authenticating strengths contributes greatly to how people perceive themselves. A technique derived from narrative therapy employs creative audiences to do just that by asking someone who is connected to the person to identify those times when the person has behaved in a way that mirrors their 'preferred identity', that is, being the best person they could be. When adopting this idea with families and/or professionals, it may be necessary to do some preparatory work as it is imperative that it doesn't become a forum for offloading what isn't going well.

CASE EXAMPLE

Burns cites the example of a woman who had a stroke when she was only 40 years old. Only able to blink initially, she still has speech difficulties two years later. She is accompanied to a hospital appointment with a friend who is asked if it surprises her that Caroline has made significant improvement. The friend replies that Caroline has always been amazing, that she's determined, stubborn, a chatterbox, remarkable. Asked if other people in her life would say that she is remarkable, Caroline says they would. (Adapted from Burns 2016, p.124)

People can be encouraged to recognise their strengths at all points of your conversation with them. This might be something as simple as responding to a person's comment about what they had been doing over the weekend. For example, someone telling you about a camping trip provides you with the opportunity to ask lots of new questions about strengths and resources: 'Did you help put up the tent?' or 'Have you done this before, or is it new?'or 'How did you work with other people to get the tent up?' Where the person is physically disabled, questions could be less about team work and more about adaptability: 'Have you slept in a tent before?' or 'What was it like, sleeping on a camp bed instead of your own one?' or 'How did you handle this?'

The more sparkling moments a person experiences – 'I did it!' moments – the more they learn to have confidence in their own abilities to meet difficult situations, and the more resilient they become. As we mentioned earlier, these sorts of conversations provide a balance for those people who are overwhelmed with failure; however, some people have been thought about negatively for long periods of time so deficiencies may need to be addressed before competences can be highlighted.

Turning deficits into strengths

Diagnoses are only helpful to people when they point very clearly to a solution: for example, someone who has appendicitis needs an appendectomy. Diagnoses can be helpful because they provide an explanation for the person's condition or behaviour and access to resources, such as a disability welfare benefit. When there is no clear solution, or a number of possible ones, diagnoses can impact negatively on people. Where someone has become burdened by a diagnosis to the point at which they stop trying and lose belief in themselves, it can be useful to turn that diagnosis on its head. For example, the Finnish psychiatric team of Furman and Ahola (1992) coined the term 'latent joy' as an alternative diagnosis for someone who is depressed by their depression.

Talking in this way with people can help both the person and the carers discover hidden strengths. For example, when someone comments that they are 'stupid', instead of reassuring them that they are not and all they need to do is work harder, you could ask, 'Are you really stupid?' or 'How stupid are you?' They are likely to reply that they are not stupid, or only a bit, at which point you become curious about the gap in perception between the person and others: 'So, if you're not that stupid, how come nobody has noticed when you are being clever?' Then you can have a fascinating conversation about how the person has come to be suffering from 'hidden cleverness', and what skills the person has that enables them to keep their cleverness secret, and how these skills can be used to help in a solution.

PRACTICE ACTIVITY

Tony was a medical orderly in the army. Whilst serving in Afghanistan, he lost both his legs in an explosion that hit his living quarters. He is being rehabilitated at a specialist army facility prior to returning home to his wife and two young sons. Never having been particularly sporty, he is depressed at the culture of superhero challenges many of the other men in the unit are planning. Neither can he see any future for himself as a husband and father. He tells you that he is useless:

- How could you have a conversation with Tony that focuses on usefulness?

Special abilities

Disabled children often have special abilities that exist in the realms of intuition, imagination or wizardry, or specific talents, such as music, so it is important to search for these abilities by entering the person's world of imagination with them. We ask people what special abilities they have that they keep secret. For many children, this is an ability to keep their feelings secret, an ability to look sad when they are not particularly sad and vice versa. Another way to access special abilities is to ask a child what character they are most like in a favourite book, film or television series. *Harry Potter* is an excellent resource for disabled children as the books are full of characters with special abilities. Or you could ask non-conforming people what their unique qualities are that help them survive at school or home without conforming. For lots of creative ideas and questions, see Freeman *et al.* (1997).

PRACTICE ACTIVITY

- Think of a person you find challenging to work with now. Now think of three good things about this person.

- What difference will recognising these good things make to your work with that person?

- Does the person know these good things about themselves?

- What questions can you ask the person that will reveal these things about them?

Resilience in workers

It is not necessarily the people you help who are the major challenge to the people's workforce. Constant organisational changes and upheavals, impending staff cutbacks, more directives from government guidance and stressful meetings all take their toll on even the most enthusiastic worker. So, you, too, need an awareness of your strengths and resources so that you can stay resilient. We end this chapter with an exercise designed to help you begin that process.

PRACTICE ACTIVITY

- Make a list of the things that a professional worker in your field does that tell you that that person is good at their job.

- Do you do these things: not at all; sometimes; most of the time; always?

- Think about the things that you do sometimes.

- When do you do these?

- What is happening when you do them?

- When was the last time you did them?

- How can you do more of them so that tomorrow you are doing them for most of the time?

Key points

- As is clearly evident in this and previous chapters, an underlying theme which runs through solution focused practice is the identification of strengths that are unique to each individual. These strengths can then be utilised to tackle or work against the difficulties that people are experiencing.

- It is recognised that people tackle the same problem in different ways; likewise, people will be affected to different degrees when experiencing similar problems and difficulties. In this situation, we find that strengths talk is helpful in building up a young person's resilience.

- When identifying strengths, it is important to gain a bigger picture of how a person has specifically applied these strengths in their achievements instead of simply offering affirmation, which could close down conversation on what could otherwise be a very empowering moment for the person.

Chapter Six

Scaling Goals, Progress and Safety

One of the most practical, accessible and creative techniques of solution focused work is the asking of scaled questions. Scaled questions enable people to locate where they are in relation to their problem or goal at that particular time; to reflect on how they have got to that particular point; to set realistic and achievable goals for the next hour, day, week and month; and then to measure their progress in achieving these goals. This chapter explains how scaled questions can be used in conversations to explore future hopes and to measure what progress has been made. We also look at how scaled questions can be used to assess safety in instances where there are serious concerns about people's well-being. We use case examples from our experience and provide activities to illustrate how these techniques can be used within very different and varied contexts.

Building relationships

We find scaled questions attractive because they are so versatile and can be used in any situation, whatever the context. They help in building therapeutic relationships because they focus on the problem in a way that separates it from the person, reduces embarrassment and shame, and allows humour to creep into the conversation. There are no template scales that work for everyone; the key is to find the particular technique that works for each individual person, enabling them to explore where they are in relation to the number, shape or character with which they have identified.

It is essential to remember that where somebody positions themselves is unique to them; there is no set of universal characteristics or defined agenda that says that if you place yourself at 4 you will have achieved xyz. For example, if you ask an ill person to locate the severity of their pain on a scale of 1–10 (where 1 = no pain and 10 = the worst pain), an answer of 9 does not necessarily mean that the person is suffering more than a person who gives an answer of 5 (with the inference that the former person needs more pain relief than the latter). It may simply mean that the person with the high score has medium pain, but it has become so chronic that they are being more badly affected than before; whilst the lower-scoring person may have acute pain but feel able to bear it because it is a transient pain. The ratings will mean more if you devise pain scales that are relevant to *each person's situation.*

Solution focused scaling recognises, and works with, the subjectivity of each person's scale, and it is useful to think of this as a process that is interested in the relationship between scores, rather than fixing on a specific score. For example, if someone tells you that their situation is currently 4 (where 1 is bad and 10 is the best), then this will mean something to them and may indicate something to you. This does not provide much material for change, however, whereas asking someone the further question about what 5 looks like will provide clues for moving forward. The difference between 4 and 5 is the space for ideas for change

Generally, we have found it useful to phrase scaled questions so that the problem is more severe towards the bottom of the scale and problem resolution towards the top as generally people seem to prefer to go up a scale rather than down. Follow-on questions, such as, 'What will be happening differently when you are at 6 on this scale?' are key to developing change.

CASE EXAMPLE

Despite having a learning disability, Jason lives in a one-bedroom flat, supported by a daily visit from a team of carers. He has begun to experience increasingly frequent epileptic seizures, which are causing his carers serious concern for his safety. He has not been keeping to his medication regime and this has made the seizures more likely, leading to concerns that Jason cannot continue to live independently.

Jason was asked to rate on a smiley face 1–10 scale how good he was at remembering to take his lamotrigine and he rated himself at 5. He was asked if he had ever been at 6 and he remembered that he had been better at taking his medication a few weeks previously. This was confirmed by the carers. Jason and his carers were asked what had been happening differently then and they were able to recall that they had talked about the medication at breakfast, which seemed to set him on the right course for the rest of the day. It was agreed that there would be 'meds-talk' every morning and that as an experiment this could be done by phone to see if this would also work for Jason.

Although a typical scale is a numerical one of 0–10, with 0 being the worst things can get and 10 being the best, we have used wider scales of 0–100, or more, depending on what has most meaning and use for people. We rather like this, as it allows for some fun and creativity, plus it allows the person to bring their individual 'twist' to the process. Sometimes, people go way off the margins we initially set; for example, minus 50 (life is dreadful) or 3 zillion (life is brilliant), but we generally just go along with this as the principle is about using the relationships between scores rather than being stuck on a scale, so follow-up questions would include:

- How come it's not lower than 50?

- What would minus 49 look like?

- What did you do to get to 3 zillion?

- What will be happening at 4 zillion?

It is possible to develop scales that are made up of shapes which start small and gradually get larger or start large and get smaller so that a person can indicate the size of the problem without actually talking about the problem. This can be helpful where people are struggling to talk about a difficult problem or because of their communication styles. We have also used pictures or characters at either end of the scale. These can be tailored to fit the understanding of the person and offer up opportunities for conversation; for example, deciding what animal might represent a calm state of mind (a sloth, an elephant) and which might be the most volatile (a tiger, a Tasmanian devil) can be quite fun. The person can then be invited to locate themselves on a scale between the two, and then consider where they would like to be, perhaps choosing another animal to represent this.

A Norwegian health care company helped young people manage their illness better by using the metaphor of a turtle (slow but long-lived) captaining a ship. The person is then invited to consider that although they are disabled, they are still captain of their own ship and need the crew (the professionals) to do what the captain needs them to do (Gerd.Nysethen@helse-nordtrondelag.no). The conversation would then be able to move into how they will achieve this change.

A technique that we have found useful is to use scales drawn on larger pieces of paper – or preferably stiff card – placing the numbers on the floor so that people can place themselves next to them. This is especially useful when working with groups of people, although do take care to allow sufficient room between each number to prevent crowding, especially with groups of wheelchair users.

Scaled questions for commitment to change

We all like to be helpful so we have a habit of giving advice, even when not asked for it. This is not a good idea until you have worked out whether or not a person needs advice – and considers you credible enough to listen to your advice. It may well be part of your job to educate people on a range of health issues, such as smoking cessation, healthy eating, managing diabetes, resistance to substance misuse and so on; however, we find that while people are perfectly aware of the dangers associated with their health issues, they often view them as too distant to be relevant. They know all about calories and healthy diets, but still love junk food. And they often know a lot more about their medical condition than you do. They are more likely to share this knowledge with you when you talk about risk-taking behaviours in a way that is meaningful to them, and not merely as a list of the negatives. People are more likely to be motivated to do something about their problems if they feel you have their best interests at heart, accept their goals, respect their views and pay attention to their wishes.

Of course, there will be times when you can't accept their goals because they are harmful to the person and/or other people. In these cases, it is helpful to assess the person's motivation for change by working out whether it is a situation of 'can't do' or 'won't do'. There are three simple scales which are very helpful here:

- If 1 is you can't be bothered to do anything about your problem and 10 is you would do anything it takes, where are you on this scale right now?

- If 1 is you have no confidence in your ability to do anything about your problem and 10 is you are completely confident, where are you on this scale right now?

- If 1 is you haven't a clue what to do about your problem and 10 is you know exactly what you need to do, where are you on this scale right now?

As can be seen from these scales, the first tests the person's motivation, or determination, to change, the second tests ability and the third knowledge. Your advice could be needed if the person gave a low rating to the third question, but not necessarily as there are follow-up questions to be asked first. Supposing a person rated themselves at 6 on the first scale, 4 on the second and 2 on the third; a logical follow-up question would be directed to the third question answer: 'What will you be doing differently when you are at 2½ or 3 on this scale?' You can also ask exception questions: 'Can you remember a time when you had a higher score? What were you doing differently then?' or 'What will people notice differently about you when you are a point higher?' Your advice comes in useful *only* after the person has worked out what help and resources they require from you. Asking these scaled questions helps you assess and develop willingness, confidence and capacity to change without you having to get into labelling people as uncooperative, useless, manipulative and so on, and without the sullen stand-offs that sometimes occur between even the most well-meaning worker and seemingly recalcitrant person when both have become pessimistic about the possibility of change.

Consider that you are working with someone who is trying to stop smoking. You could ask them, 'If I have a stopping smoking success scale of 1–10, where 1 is you are nowhere near ready to stop and 10 is you couldn't be better motivated, where are you on this scale?' Once the person has identified where they are on the scale, you would then enquire about how they got to place themselves there and what has happened to make them think that this was their scale. The person may say that they are at 7 because they have tried and succeeded to stop before, or that they are motivated by friends stopping, or that they have been given a health warning.

The next stage is to identify what steps the person thinks would be helpful to them, whether this is something that they can achieve or if someone else can help them move up the scale. Small steps to get up the scale are explored, as the assumption is that big changes are not necessarily required. It is also acknowledged that progress is not necessarily consistent, with some people taking large steps and making huge progress, whereas others may need to stay at the same number for a while and continue to work at what has been going well. They can look at moving forward after some period of consistency has been achieved. The important issue is to be led by what the person identifies is best for them. Talking with them about their ideas for how *they* are going to move forward can increase levels of self-belief, responsibility taking, ownership and autonomy.

So, referring back to our example of identifying what else could be happening to move one point further up the scale to achieve their goal, the smoker may identify that they might also need to reduce their coffee intake, find something to do with their hands when they get the urge to smoke, let smoking friends know that they are stopping, or just be more determined. Rayya Ghul said that for her:

> *When I finally gave up cigarettes I found that the strategy that worked best for me was to think 'what would a non-smoker do?' every time I had an urge to smoke. I hit on it because I was trying to think back to something in my past which would prove I could do something I thought was impossible. I remembered that I had really struggled to learn to drive and was convinced that I would never be able to. Then I thought to myself, there are an awful lot of people who drive and I can't be that different to them. I passed my driving test a few weeks later. Then I applied it to smoking. I had always had excuses for why I needed a cigarette. However, there are a lot of people who manage their lives perfectly well without reaching for a cigarette. I became curious. What did they do instead? (2015, p.96)*

The key is that these are ideas that the person has thought of *for themselves* which they believe will work for them. This means that it is highly unlikely, even though you may work with people in similar contexts, that the ideas/tasks that they come up with will be the same. This is why it is difficult to provide a 'script' for solution focused therapeutic conversations – their direction depends entirely on the local ideas, strengths and solutions of that particular person.

CASE EXAMPLE

Claire has recently found it difficult to eat, particularly in company. She has lost some weight and is beginning to withdraw from the activities she enjoyed.

Therapist: So where would you put yourself on the scale today?

Claire: About 2.

Therapist: Have you ever felt lower than 2?

Claire: Yeah, I've been as low as 0.

Therapist: That sounds pretty bad... How did you get yourself to 2?

Claire: My friends helped, talking to them... They kept an eye on me.

Therapist: So you enlisted the help of your friends to get up to 2. That's clever, I wonder what would life look like at a 3.

Claire: [thinks for a while] I'd be eating a little more.

Therapist: Eating a little more would get you up the scale a little. What do you think you'd be able to eat?

Claire: A piece of fruit.

Therapist: Sounds like a good start. When would you be able to eat that?

Claire: When others are having their lunch.

Therapist: Would you eat it with your friends?

Claire: I suppose I could, yes.

Therapist: What kind of fruit will you be eating?

Claire: Some grapes or an apple...

Therapist: What would that feel like?

Claire: I'll start to feel a bit more normal...eating when they do.

Therapist: That sounds a little bit like your miracle day, eating something with your friends... How likely is it that, between now and when we next meet, you will be able to eat a piece of fruit? Say 0 is not at all likely, 10 is you definitely will do it...

Claire: Very likely... I think I'd be an 8 or 9.

(Adapted from Jacob 2001, pp.25–26)

PRACTICE ACTIVITIES

1. On a confidence scale of 1–10, where 1 is not at all and 10 is completely, how confident are you about using a solution focused approach with the people with whom you work?

   • Make a list of the follow-up questions you need to ask yourself next.

2. Think of a project you are involved with (such as landscaping your garden, dieting, completing a course of study) and ask yourself the following questions:

   • If 0 is you haven't even started your project and 10 is you have satisfactorily completed it, where are you on this scale?

   • On a scale of 0–10, how satisfied are you with your score?

   • When you are one point higher on the scale, what will you be doing differently?

   • Where do you think (partner, colleagues, friends) would put you on the scale?

   • What will you be doing differently that will tell that person you are higher on the scale? What else?

   • What did you do to get to your score? What else?

   • Does this indicate that you have the resources and skills needed to complete the project?

   • What resources and skills do you have that you are not yet using in your efforts to complete the project?

   • Are there any resources you need to acquire in order to complete the project?

- What is the first small step you could take to achieve your goal?

Remember that a big project like landscaping your garden will take time and that you may be happy with small, regular achievements. Equally, you may not wish to ever get to 10; gardens can be lifetime projects.

3. With a group of colleagues, think of a hobby or sport you currently engage in and at which you would like to be better. Set out a scale of 1–10 along the floor, where 1 is you are regularly performing as badly as you can imagine and 10 is you are consistently performing at your personal peak. Everyone places themselves on the scale. Then discuss with person nearest to you:

- How did you get to this point?

- What does 10 represent?

- Where would you like to be?

- What do you need to do to get you to this point?

- What help will you require?

- Who would be best placed to help you?

- What time scale will be reasonable for you to achieve your goal?

Scaled questions for discovering people's hopes and wishes

If people are to move into a problem-free future, then it is helpful to know what their aspirations are and help them achieve these. People can experience lives that are so full of defeat and despair, however, that it is difficult for them to have any aspirations, as the way they have been raised or the ways that society has treated them can create a sense of hopelessness or they may have conditions that, whilst not directly life-threatening, take away their zest for life and sap their energy: unpleasant symptoms, lack of mobility, being unable to return to work or restart a hobby, feeling isolated and alone, beginning to blame oneself or become angry that there is no magic cure.

Workers with people with chronic incurable conditions move away from talking about 'cure' so that the person can explore other options, take more responsibility for their well-being, and stop searching for an elusive cure (Craggs-Hinton 2015; Burns 2016). There is evidence that moving from the search for a magic cure to more positive thoughts leads to a better outcome for young people with chronic fatigue syndrome (Crawley et al 2017).

The process by which people come to acceptance and rediscover hope can be speeded up by the careful use of scaled questions. Scaled questions also reveal unexpected acceptance and hope.

CASE EXAMPLE

Francis is 80. He has advanced prostate and bone cancer, and has been referred for help with his swallowing as he is only managing to eat drink and very small amounts. Having done a swallowing assessment and discussed soft-consistency food that Francis could choose from the menu, the therapist decides to ask him a scaling question:

Therapist: On a scale of 0–10, with 0 being things aren't too good and 10 being things are going pretty well, where would you say you are generally now?

Francis: About 2.

Therapist: So...I know you've been in hospital for a while, and things aren't much fun being stuck in hospital. You could have told me 0. How have you managed to be at a number 2?

Francis: It's about getting out there and doing it. I've been trying to keep myself occupied.

Therapist: What are you doing to keep yourself occupied? Do you listen to the hospital radio or watch television?

Francis: No. I don't like the radio or television. I sometimes write. See if you can find a red notebook over there...

It transpires that Francis has written a very funny piece on 'The hospital gown and hospital beds'.

(Adapted from Burns 2016, p.36)

Scaled questions are also useful when working with people who deny that they have a problem or aren't bothered by it.

PRACTICE ACTIVITY

An extremely fit young man who played football and cricket to a high standard and liked to go drinking with his friends at weekends, Jim was diagnosed with diabetes at 19. After being stabilised and trained how to administer his insulin injections, Jim was left to pick up the pieces of his life. He played a furiously fought football match, followed by a night out with his mates, resulting in him collapsing and being rushed to hospital. Despite knowing how to manage his diabetes, Jim continued with unsuitable old habits. For example, as he has never eaten between meals, he does not always carry some carbohydrate with him when out. He easily becomes hypoglycaemic, which makes him even more uncooperative when his girlfriend urges him to eat. (Adapted from Shone 2013, pp.6–8)

- What scaled questions could you ask Jim?

Hint: We find that the most effective questions are those that 'click' with the person, perhaps by having a particular meaning for them, and stimulate them into thinking about changing their situation.

- Thinking of Jim's sporting prowess and ability to restrict his eating, what metaphors might have meaning for Jim?

Scaled questions for managing feelings

People can often find it difficult to talk about their feelings, sometimes because they have been brought up not to do so or because they are overwhelmed by the strength of those feelings. They can also choose not to discuss their feelings because they are unsure about whether they can handle them or simply because they consider them to be personal and private.

Scaled questions can help people to identify and express their feelings by providing a graded and nuanced framework that avoids binary or general answers. Just asking someone how they feel can lead to stock answers such as 'Good,' 'Fine' or 'Bad,' which aren't really telling us much about what they are actually feeling, and lack detail about the complexities of their emotions. Asking someone to place their feelings on a scale invites them to think about where they would locate them and why this would be at a particular number rather than any other, enabling them to reflect on the detail of their feelings and go through a process of comparison with times when this has been worse and/or better. This opens up opportunities to be curious and ask questions about what led them to place themselves at that number, which then enables further conversations about what would have to be happening differently for it to be less of a problem. Solution focused practice accepts that people have feelings and that these are often not within their control; however, how people 'do' feelings through their behaviour is manageable and able to change, so we are interested in how people might behave differently when these feelings happen again.

We live in a society that is full of advice about emotional states, how to talk about them and what to do to make people feel better. A cursory glance at magazines, newspaper articles, social media and online websites will find discussions about how to understand yourself through popular psychology and the latest counselling terminology to describe your personality, feelings and relationship styles. You can even complete self-assessments that tell you what 'type' of person you are and what this means for your life. The result is that people often describe their lives, thoughts and feelings in ways that reflect the stories that are around them, and this has consequences when working with people. For example, when people come to see us, they often say that their problem is their low self-esteem, a frequently used concept. Self-esteem is a complex idea, however, and, rather than it being a fixed state of being, it can vary from day to day depending on the context people are in. It can even be both high and low at the same time as different aspects of self-esteem are considered; for example, a person might be feeling worthless in a work situation but full of confidence when cooking a meal.

A solution focused approach asks questions about self-esteem to encourage detail and reduce the totalising label placed on such feelings, using scaling questions to help the person choose which parts of their self-esteem can be changed for the better. For example, we might ask the person, 'If 0 is the worst person you can be, and 100 the best, where would you rate yourself on this scale today?' A follow-up question could be, 'On a scale of 0–10, how satisfied are you with your score?' and then, 'What will you be doing differently when you are at a point higher?'

PRACTICE ACTIVITY

- Make a list of the things a professional people worker does that tells you they are good at their job.

- Scale yourself about whether you do these things: not at all; sometimes; most of the time; always.

- Think about the things you do *sometimes*.

- When do you do these?

- What is happening when you do them?

- When was the last time you did them?

- How can you do more of them so that tomorrow you are doing them *most of the time*?

We find that with solution focused practice it is important not to rush your questions, giving the person plenty of time to think, and to begin thinking deeply. By moving too quickly, you can close down thinking and steer the conversation in your preferred direction, rather than the person's. Asking people to really think about their situation and to work to find their solutions is actually very demanding and people often find it quite exhausting. We recognise this by asking questions such as:

- You've worked hard today; on a scale of 0–10, how has it been for you?

- So that we can make the best of our next session, what would have made it a little better?

- After all today's hard work, how are you going to treat yourself this evening?

These sorts of questions are important not only because we want to make sure that we are on the right track for the person, but also because we want them to begin looking at what techniques they have for looking after themselves. This can give us clues about their preferences, hopes, desires and potential solutions.

We have found that some people are subjected to unreasonable demands, either by others or by themselves through their upbringing or social situation. For example, where someone has a disability, demands on carers, which seemed reasonable in the beginning, gradually and chronically creep into all areas of family life, as Brown and Brown confirm:

The more complex the disability, the more likely it is that family life will become increasingly oriented around the needs of the person with the disability. When this occurs, family members do not have as much time available for social, productive, leisure or spiritually oriented activities, and this very often impacts negatively on family quality of life. (2003, p.191)

The carer may resent the way in which their responsibilities have increased but feel unable to do anything about it in case they are seen as uncaring or selfish. Here we would ask questions such as:

- Suppose we have a 'responsibility taking' scale where 0 is you take some responsibility and 10 is you take all the responsibility for what happens in your family. Where on this scale would you place yourself?

- On a scale from 0–10, how achievable do you think is this responsibility taking?

- On a scale of 0–10, what do you think would be a reasonable score for the circumstances in which you are living?

We would also talk about being 'sensibly selfish' so that the person remains emotionally and physically strong, developing a plan where the responsibility taken is both reasonable and achievable.

CASE EXAMPLE

When her mother began to have minor heart attacks, Marie moved to a house nearby in a small village. Her eldest son, Daniel, moved in with her after his relationship broke down, and she supervises his contact with his baby son to guard against his ex-partner's accusations of neglect. She shops, cooks and cleans for her mother, tasks which are made difficult by her father's verbal abuse. He has always been aggressive towards both Marie and her mother, favouring his younger daughter, Sandra. His aggression is unpredictable as he is becoming increasingly demented. Her younger son, Damien, and his partner, Emma, who live many miles away, have recently had a baby boy who required special baby care after a difficult birth. Marie has been visiting Damien fortnightly to help out and the couple have asked her to babysit two days a week so that Emma can return to work.

Marie's husband, Milton, has been feeling increasingly tired and depressed and has now been diagnosed with amyloidosis. There are no treatment options for him, other than a drastic reduction in his fluid intake. Marie is desperate for a break and has suggested taking Milton to a spa hotel where he can lounge by the pool but he lacks the energy or will to do this, spending most of each day sitting on the sofa.

Marie rated herself well over the end of a 'responsibility taking' scale, launching into a bitter account of the lack of help she receives from her sister. She wasn't sure where on the 'responsibility taking' she would like to be or what would be reasonable and achievable, so she was asked more scaled questions about responsibility taking for each member of her family. She thought that a score of 2 was reasonable and achievable responsibility taking for her parents (because her sister could do more and her father didn't appreciate her efforts, anyway); 7 for her husband (his brother and large circle of male friends could do more, and Milton could supervise Daniel's contact with his son as he was always in the room, albeit on the sofa), and 9 for Damien and Emma and their baby boy (because they had no social support).

Marie decided to stay with Damien and Emma for two to three days each week despite the lengthy travel as this was a caring responsibility she enjoyed and took her away from responsibilities at home that she didn't enjoy, or find achievable. She was confident that her sister, elder son and Milton's brother and friends could pick up the rest of the responsibility taking.

Not all scaled questions go from 0–10; as in the first question above, it makes more sense to reverse the numbers. The key issue is to ensure that everyone is clear what the scales mean. It is important to remember which way round you ask your scales and it can help if you draw the scale on a piece of paper with the 'meanings' written at each end. Not only are these drawings useful for your records, but they are a visual reminder for the person's progress at later sessions. Scales can also be incorporated into feedback notes. Using a format adapted from Berg and Reuss (1998), we separate a person's progress (what they have done) from solutions (how they did it), as shown in the following case example. We also take care to use the person's own words.

CASE EXAMPLE

Name: Melvyn

Date: 26 October

Problem

Melvyn has made a lot of progress in solving his problems. On a scale where 0 is how the problem was at the beginning and 10 is the problem is completely solved, Melvyn is at 6 or 7, sometimes even 8. At other times, he has less good days and slips to 4. He would like to have more confidence, be less intense, have control over his drinking and have a better social life.

Progress

1. Melvyn has got to 6 or 7 on the problem solved scale by managing work stresses better, and not letting his boss put his work stresses onto him.

2. Drinking had got really bad (two bottles each night and hiding one of them from his family) but Melvyn hasn't had a drink since Saturday. He feels a lot better for this.

3. He has had some good days when he's met up with friends and had a laugh.

4. Melvyn can remember a time when he had confidence and was funny.

Solutions

1. Melvyn handles work stress by working out what the worst is that could happen to the business and dealing with things day to day. He has become expert in negotiating with suppliers who are pressing for payment and/or interest. He used to work, work, work but now he recognises when he's done all he can. He also takes time out at work to see a friend, which helps with stress levels, and makes up any time needed at weekends. To stop his boss putting his stress onto him, Melvyn simply explained to him what he could do and what he wasn't going to do.

2. There has been no drinking since Saturday because it became more bother than it was worth to lie about the other bottle of wine. And Melvyn just decided that he didn't like being controlled by drink.

3. The good days have included meeting old friends, deciding on a hobby he and his mate Ben can do together (maybe fishing) and spending some time with his other mate Jim. Melvyn has also been asked to holiday in Canada by a girl he shares an email relationship with.

4. The times when Melvyn had confidence and was funny were when he had a social circle, like at university. He enjoyed having a circle of friends to do things with and the opportunities to meet new people who joined the circle.

Next steps

1. Melvyn has lots of options – maybe get an apartment, move back to London, start university again and so on – so, he will give his options more consideration and see which one suits him most.

2. He might toss a coin each day and pretend to be confident and funny when it comes up heads. If it comes up tails, he can have an ordinary day. He can see how these days feel.

3. He might try some new stuff to see what sorts of hobbies suit him and have the most promising social circles.

4. As Melvyn can get himself out of bad patches within two days, he might notice how he does this. He must be doing right at these times because, before, his life was consistently shitty.

As solutions often come from asking what the person will be doing 'instead' when the problem has gone, it is helpful to construct scales which ask people to rate themselves on the behaviours which are natural opposites to undesirable behaviours. A person who appears to be indifferent to the feelings of others can be asked scaled questions about caring and thoughtfulness, whilst one who responds to feelings of unhappiness with depressive behaviours – lack of appetite, confidence, lack of energy and so on – can be asked to scale themselves on a happiness scale. This typically would consist of, 'If 0 is life as miserable as it could possibly get and 100 is the sun is shining and you couldn't be happier, where are you on this scale?' This is followed up with scaled questions about how satisfied the person is with their rating. They may be very satisfied as they may be doing as well as could be expected in very difficult circumstances, in which case you would ask questions about how they are coping and what qualities they are using. For the more likely situation where a person is not satisfied with their rating, you would ask where on the scale they would like to be and how they could get there.

It is also useful to have a conversation about how they will 'do happiness'. People often say things like, 'I'd be smiling, I'd just be happier,' whereas if you asked them how they do misery, they will have a detailed list of behaviours: cry a lot, say no when my friends ask me out, go off my food, can't sleep and so on. A close examination of 'doing happiness' with a person will reveal the behaviours which have a happy meaning for that person. These usually consist of doing various activities which give them a sense of achievement and of being valued, and often involve loved ones, so you ask questions such as:

- As well as laughing more, what else will you be doing when you are happier?

- What will you be doing when you are back to your 'bubbly' self?

- What will you be doing that would make me, your partner and your children realise that you are happier?

- How would anyone else notice that you are happier?

Similar scaled questions can be used for situations where the person is tense and anxious.

CASE EXAMPLE

We met Sam in Chapter 2 (see pp.42–43), where he was anxious about his forthcoming operation. After establishing that 'being less anxious', which he described as 'Jangly Nerves', was his goal, the nurse continues with scaled questions:

Jane: Okay, so it sounds like what you want is to feel more in control of the Jangly Nerves. Let's look at these Jangly Nerves in closer detail. On a scale of 1–10 (one being least, 10 being worst) how would you rate those Jangly Nerves now?

Sam: I'd say 6.

Jane: And where on the scale would you like to be, so that you have felt calm and okay.

Sam: Ice. I'd say a 4 would look good.

Jane: All right 4 would be good. And how would 5 feel?

Sam: If I could get to feeling 5 by the end of today, then that would be a great start.

Jane: Yes, I agree, it really would. So let's talk about those Jangly Nerves some more. Sam, when do they seem more obvious, more out there?

Sam: I have no idea. They're always there.

Jane: Well, suppose I asked your wife to answer that question. What you think she'd say?

Sam: That's easy, she'd say it's whenever something happens that might take me away from always being in charge. She says I just hate it when things happen that I can't control.

Jane: Oh, that's interesting. So now, I wonder what your wife would say you are like when you are calm. Do you think she'd be able to think of times when your Jangly Nerves are not so apparent.

Sam: She'd probably say I'm calm when I've had a holiday, when I'm lying in my hammock reading a detective story. As a matter of fact those are some times when I'm quite okay.

Jane: So, suppose a miracle happened overnight, and the Jangly Nerves just went away. What would you be doing and feeling, can you describe that to me?

Sam: I'd be cool, calm, collected, able to go into that surgery knowing that I was doing the right thing, and pretty much accepting of the surgeon's skills.

Jane: Maybe if we tried using some of the cool, calmness that seems to come out when you are lying in that hammock, and applying it to this situation, your Jangly Nerves might be less obvious. What do you think?

Sam: Well, I'm willing to give it a try...

(McAllister 2007, pp.41–42)

PRACTICE ACTIVITY

- Choose a person with whom you are working who has difficulty controlling their emotions.

- Devise a scale that is appropriate to their particular difficulties and ask them to rate themselves on it. Be creative.

- Should the person look at you in bewilderment, ask the person what would be a better a scale for them.

Scaled questions for assessing safety

Scaled questions are especially useful in safeguarding situations as they enable you to give people the opportunity to express their views and participate in decisions that affect them even when the situations they are in are dangerous. Scaled questions can be devised for any safety situation, from safety in crossing the road, to safety in serious safeguarding situations. They have in common the key question of how risk can be reduced and safety developed, measured and demonstrated.

So, for example, if you are concerned about someone's binge drinking, you could ask, 'On a Saturday safe good night out scale, if 1 is you are likely to be upside down in a flower bed at 2 o'clock and 10 is by 2 o'clock you will be in a taxi going home and have managed to tell the driver your correct address, where are you on this scale today?' Or where you are concerned about a person's reluctance to give themselves an insulin injection, you could ask, 'On a getting over my embarrassment about injecting where people might see me scale, if 1 is you would definitely miss an injection and 10 is you would just do it whoever was about, where are you on this scale today?' Or where you are worried about a person who has difficulty in eating, you could ask, 'On a scale of 1–10, where 1 is there's not a snowball's chance in hell you'd eat a lettuce leaf and 10 is you'd definitely eat fish, chips and pudding, where are you on this scale today?' This latter question is one of many wonderful examples in Frederike Jacob's book on recovery from eating distress (2001).

Constructing scaled questions with a wide range of opposites is especially useful in serious safeguarding situations because they discourage untruthfulness and give the vulnerable person a voice. For example, by asking a person to rate their caring on a scale, where 1 is Shannon Matthews's mum and 10 is Mother Teresa (you can vary role models depending on current news stories and local contexts), you have made it clear that you do not expect them to place themselves at either extreme. It doesn't matter where they place themselves because you can still talk about what they need to be doing differently to move up the scale.

You can also ask the vulnerable person where they would scale the carer. It is unlikely the vulnerable person will give them a really low score but even a fraction of a point makes space for the person to say how they would prefer to be cared for. You can also vary the questions to allow for professional concerns to be raised without getting into an argument or a sullen stand-off. For example, a worker concerned about someone with learning disabilities neglecting themselves in their independent living could ask, 'You rate your self-care at 9 and I rate it at 2. What do you think you will be doing differently when we can both agree?' The worker might also talk about a time when they were able to rate the person's self-care higher, and ask what was happening differently, then that can be used to develop better self-care in the future. A useful question here is, 'What have you forgotten to do that was working for you before?'

Even rating someone at 2 means that they are not at 1 or 0, so there is space to talk about what is going well. This allows for ideas about how to get up the scale and what support might be helpful in getting there. It also helps the worker to be clear about what is good enough for the person to retain their independence, being very clear what 1 looks like and that this would mean they lose their independence. Equally, it is helpful to spell out what 10 looks like in detail that is specific and measurable, so that everyone is clear about what is required. These details could include the person paying their bills, being respectful of neighbours when playing music or having friends round, buying food to eat rather than too much alcohol, remembering to have a bath, cleaning the flat on a regular basis and so on. With this sort of scale, people know exactly what the worst is that could happen to them and what they need to do to avoid this worst-case scenario. It also provides them with a means of measuring progress as the scale is revisited with them.

CASE EXAMPLE

Alan has been disturbed several days before been detained under legal powers at his home. He resisted transfer by ambulance and was brought to the secure unit in handcuffs by the police. This is a section of his second interview on the unit:

Interviewer: So thinking about a scale of 0 to 10 where 10 is you're out of hospital and things are going well, and 0 is as bad as things were before, where are you right now on that scale?

Alan: Nought.

Interviewer: So how have you kept going when you are at nought?

Alan: Getting some sleep helped.

Interviewer: So sleep is really important for you. When you move up half a point on the scale what will be different for you?

Alan: I won't feel like hitting people.

Interviewer: Who did you feel like hitting?

Alan: The neighbours and that policeman. He had no right to put handcuffs on me.

Interviewer: How come the police were there?

Alan: I told the ambulance man I would cut him if he tried to come into my flat.

Interviewer: Have you cut anyone before? Or hit anyone?

Alan: No; but I would have done it.

Interviewer: How come you did not do that?

Alan: They came in before I could get a knife from the kitchen.

Interviewer: Do you still think about getting a knife for cutting someone?

Alan: I sometimes think about it.

Interviewer: How did you manage to think about it but not do it?

Alan: I think to myself that they will put me in hospital again if I cut someone. The neighbours might get me for it while I was sleeping.

Interviewer: Are there specific people that you think of cutting, neighbours or anyone else?

Alan: I felt like hitting that policeman.

Interviewer: Have you thought about cutting or hitting anyone in this hospital?

Alan: No.

Interviewer: How can we tell if you are thinking about cutting someone or hitting someone?

Alan: I don't know.

Interviewer: Will you tell us if you are thinking that?

Alan: [no reply]

Interviewer: When you're thinking like that, what can we do that will help?

Alan: Let me stay my room; the other people here are strange.

Interviewer: Will you tell us when you need to stay in your room?

Alan: Yes.

Interviewer: Okay; we will ask you if we are not sure. I guess that hitting or cutting someone would not help you get out of hospital sooner.

Alan: [nods]

Interviewer: Anything else to mention today?

Alan: No; I'm tired of talking just now.

(Adapted from Macdonald 2011, p.164)

PRACTICE ACTIVITIES

1. Imagine you are due to see Alan the following day after he has had some good-quality sleep:

   • Devise a set of scaled questions that will help Alan have a clear idea of what needs to happen for him to get out of hospital.

2. Select someone with whom you are working and where you are frustrated with their lack of cooperation:

    • With the help of at least two colleagues, construct a set of scaled questions that will allow you to begin talking about your concerns in a way that will engage their interest.

3. We were tempted to invite you to co-construct a progress chart with a person but, instead, we end this chapter with an altogether more difficult exercise. Imagine that a person you are currently working with is interviewed about the usefulness of your support/intervention. On a scale of 1–10, where 1 is it was no help at all and 10 is it was everything they could have hoped for, where do you think that person would scale your support/intervention? When you have identified where you think they would scale your intervention, consider the following:

    • What did you do to get to this score? What else?

    • How did you do it? What else?

    • What skills, abilities and qualities did you show?

    • What will be happening/different when the person scales your intervention one point up the scale?

    • What steps will you have taken to achieve this?

    • How will your skills, abilities and qualities support you in moving your work forward with the person?

Key points

• The versatility of scaled questions means that they can be applied from the beginning in both establishing goals and later in defining where someone is in relation to their goal(s), and then woven in and out of the conversation. The technique therefore fits very well with the general fluidity of the approach.

• Scaled questions are also attractive to use as they can be applied within different contexts alongside the actual scale being designed in different ways, that is, numbers and not always 1–10, shapes, people, colours and so on. The technique allows for differing opinions to be registered without causing friction, whilst subsequent questions ('Gosh, you have scaled yourself at a 10, how have you got there?') provide a platform for people to reflect and justify their original scale. We often find that when they are given this opportunity, people more often than not review their original position for a lower number. Similarly, when there are worries about a person's behaviour, it encourages and enables concerned parties, both professionals and family members, to voice where they are and, equally importantly, to provide an explanation of what they believe needs to be different to lessen those worries and move further up the scale to safety.

- We will all have been in situations when people find it extremely difficult to communicate; this can often be misconstrued and result in labels such as 'difficult', 'resistant' and 'reluctant'. Scaled questions can help to clarify a person's position about how willing they are to move forward and how confident they are in doing so. This then enables you as a worker to make an informed and collaborative assessment about their motivation and capabilities.

Chapter Seven

Bringing It All Together

This final chapter looks at how the principles, techniques and ideas from the previous chapters can be brought together in a solution focused conversation. We bring examples of how conversations can be structured and include ideas for 'homework' or follow-up tasks to be completed between sessions. Recording is a key element of formal interventions and we explore what forms this can take in a solution focused approach. Some situations can become 'stuck' or progress may be slow, so we bring some ideas on how to 'unblock' and move forward. Working with other agencies and professions is an important aspect of people work, so we provide suggestions for how this can be done successfully in a solution focused manner.

Bringing it all together

It will be clear from the previous chapters that in working with people we are interested in their ideas for solutions that make a difference. When we meet with people, we find that questions adapted from Chris Iveson's (2002, p.151) summary are helpful in keeping us focused on current resources and future hopes:

- What do you hope to achieve from our meeting?

- What will your problem-free life look like?

- What are you already doing that can help you to get there?

- How did you do that?

- What will be different when one small step is taken towards it?

Similarly, De Jong and Berg (2008, pp.17–18) describe the structure of a solution focused session as:

- Describing the problem

- Developing well-formed goals

- Exploring for exceptions

- End of session feedback

- Evaluating progress.

We find that the beauty, and difficulty, of solution focused conversations is that they are flexible and fluid around the direction in which the person wishes to go, rather than having a prescribed formula that can be restrictive, but provides boundaries. This requires discipline from the worker to follow the conversation intently to make sure that the person is being heard properly – the worker becomes a 'solution detective' (Sharry 2011), trying to find and identify any hidden or partly obscured strengths or exceptions that can assist in developing solutions.

Pre-meeting change

Most approaches to working with people assume that the 'business' takes place in the actual encounter between the worker and the person. Solution focused approaches take the view that as change always happens and the problem is rarely always happening (de Shazer 1988), it is useful when meeting someone to ask them about when the problem has been less of a problem or what steps they have taken to manage the problem, or simply what has changed. The space between the development of the problem and meeting someone to talk about it (perhaps called the referral process) can be full of ideas and experiences that can be explored and utilised to effect positive change. Solution focused workers can ask people to consider this leading up to the meeting and begin to identify those often obscured times when the problem has been actively resisted, providing a rich source of material for a conversation about solutions. Indeed, this approach can be so helpful that, sometimes, people arrive at meetings having found their own solutions and answers to their problems, and the worker is left with little to do but reinforce and assist where wanted.

This may well appear to be hopelessly optimistic, as we are culturally influenced to believe that we need to spend time supporting the person to work out their problems with our expert help, but there is evidence to support this. Talmon (1990), for example, initially presumed that those people who did not return after having had a single session of solution focused therapy were unhappy with the approach and did not want to come back for more. When he undertook follow-up research, however, he found that actually most had managed to achieve their goal and they were perfectly happy with this. Allgood *et al.* (1995) found that 30 per cent of 200 people seeking therapy reported pre-therapeutic improvement, indicating that it is worth presuming that people's situation can improve before we even meet them and therefore it is worth asking about it. Where people do experience positive change prior to formal intervention they seem to be more energised to complete therapeutic interventions – up to four times more, according to the research of Johnson, Nelson and Allgood (1998).

CASE EXAMPLE

Katy had done a lot of thinking in the period between a brief informal chat to see if the counselling service was for her and attending the first session. She arrived at her first session with her preferred solution well worked out so no assessment of her goals was undertaken; the session being used to provide her with an opportunity to identify her strengths and tell how she would 'do' her solution... Katy attended two further sessions to tell how well her solution had worked and describe how she did it in detail. Problem focused counsellors might think that the problems were insufficiently addressed and would resurface but, as solution-talk counselling has no notion of 'closure', Katy can return at any time if she needs further help.

Starting a conversation

Solution focused workers find it easy to share their understanding of people and change with those they work with, as there is no complicated theorising required to explain what is being done. Our experience tells us that many workers have theoretical perspectives (either consciously or unconsciously) which influence their judgement, practice and the outcomes for those they work with. They can often struggle to articulate these to the people with whom they are working, however, because they are over-complex or sometimes quite problematic in their assumptions about people – that there is something 'wrong' with them. We are also culturally educated to want to talk about problems and their past, so people expect that professionals will want to discuss these.

Whilst not ignoring the problems, solution focused workers can explain that their approach is 'much more interested in where they are going rather than where they have been, as the past can't be changed' (Milner and O'Byrne 2002b, p.60), and checking out with the person that this is okay with them. This gives people the option to talk about their problems, but also not to do so if they choose. People do not then feel obliged to problem talk to meet the perceived expectations of the worker. Of course, it would be disrespectful to ignore people's wish to talk about their problems, so solution focused workers will move away from problem talk as soon as is practicable and when the person has said enough to be heard.

This approach lends itself to a more solid partnership and anti-discriminatory relationship, as it is open about assumptions and processes, plus it tries to avoid imposing a theoretical framework on people and seeks to recognise the individual within the problem. Someone may well present with a problem label (drug user, schizophrenic, diabetic) that has meaning; however, we are interested in understanding the meaning of that label for that specific individual: how they experience it; how it works on them; when it is less of a problem; and so on. Pre-suppositional questions can be helpful here, those questions that contain assumptions about what has already happened. For example, rather than asking, 'Has there been a time when you have successfully dealt with the problem?' it can be made more active by asking, 'When have you successfully dealt with the problem?' The difference is that the second question presumes that someone has already done this and invites detail, whereas the first question invites a simple yes/no answer. This assists in looking for exceptions to the problem, but goes counter to some interviewing approaches that suggest the need for open-ended questioning. We believe that all our conversations with people should have the purpose of finding solutions, so, if using such questioning techniques is helpful, then we are happy to use them.

The solution focused worker will regularly ask whether the conversation is useful to the person and invite them to comment on the worker's understanding of the situation. We have found the following types of question to be helpful in doing this:

- How is this conversation going for you?

- Should we keep talking about this or would you be more interested in...?

- Is this interesting to you? Is this what we should spend time talking about?

- I was wondering if you would be more interested in me asking some more about this or whether we should focus on...?

- Am I on the right lines with these questions?

- What would we be talking about if I was being more helpful?

- What question haven't I asked that you wish I had?

- On a scale of 1–10, where 1 is this conversation has been an utter waste of time and 10 is it couldn't have been better, where would you rate it?

- If you had scored the session one point higher, what would I have been doing differently?

- If you had scored this session one point higher, what would you have been doing differently?

(Milner and Bateman 2011, pp.146–147)

PRACTICE ACTIVITY

The next time you interview someone, at the end of the session ask them, 'On a scale of 0–10, where 0 is really awful and 10 is the best it could have been, how would you rate this interview? If you were able to rate it one point higher, what would you have been doing differently?'

Records and recording

This transparency is continued by explaining to people that any notes that are taken in any meeting will be given to them to check for accuracy. This not only helps with understanding the person's perspective correctly but also engages them in the process, providing an opportunity to take some control and work together in partnership. Writing down what someone says without interpretation or editing is a useful solution focused approach that avoids losing the person's perspective and replacing it with the worker's. Using the words, terms and metaphors that the person uses is helpful, as their use of these will be meaningful for them and is a clearer expression of what they want to say, rather than changing these into professional language. It also demonstrates that we are taking them seriously.

The worker will have been seeking exceptions and strengths through their questioning and this will be reflected in the recording, providing a written record of clues for developing solutions that the person can see. This is helpful for some people who struggle to recognise any of their strengths, or view their problem as completely overwhelming, as it can reinforce the exceptions discussed in the conversation.

Sometimes, the organisation that you work with requires information to be collected and collated in certain ways. Milner and O'Byrne (2002b) developed a structure that covers areas that are usually required and is also helpful for reflection. There are four sections to this: problem description; exceptions and progress (what the person did); thoughts and solutions (how they did it); and tasks to be done (next steps forward). As solution focused work is relentlessly practical, other elements can be added if and when necessary.

CASE EXAMPLE

The following are the case notes for Michael written by Steve.

Dear Michael

As promised, here is your copy of the notes. I hope that I have got everything right but I'm not sure that I have got the sequence of the irrational fears exactly in the correct order. If I have got it wrong, please let me know next time we meet so that I can make any necessary alterations to the notes.

I hope you are impressed with yourself when you read the notes. You have achieved an enormous amount under the most extreme difficulties. This says a lot about you as a person.

Problem description

Michael has been troubled with irrational fears and obsessional thoughts. These have led to him moving out of his flat, sleeping rough, going into a hostel, and giving up his job. His family haven't been supportive in a way that would really help and this has left Michael with feelings of anger, resentment and rejection. He used to be well off but has also been very poor, and it is important to him to turn his life round and get some sort of balance. Being relaxed and getting a nice house to live in are more important than getting another job for Michael at the moment.

Exceptions and progress

1. His irrational fears and obsessional thoughts have been as high as 9 on a scale of 0–10 (where 0 is not at all and 10 is the most they can be) but they are much lower at the moment, about 6. He even handled his mother coming round to the house without too much difficulty.

2. He is still vulnerable to hurt and feels resentful but lots of the angriness has subsided.

3. He has started doing self-care and learning how to relax himself. This stops him feeling anxious all the time and his support worker has noticed a big difference in just one month. Before he talked quickly, was hunched up and couldn't look people in the eye. Now his body is much more relaxed and calm about things.

4. He only feels 2 on a scale of 0–10 (where 0 is absolutely the pits and 10 is the best he could be) good about himself but he can remember a time when he was 17 and had a much higher opinion of himself. This competent self is still there – he wouldn't have handled his difficulties and achieved so much otherwise.

Thoughts on solutions

1. He handled his first set of irrational fears about solvents, which gave him panic attacks and chest pains, by changing his job. Then his fears changed shape and he became afraid of UV rays coming through the floor of the flat he was living in, which was over a tanning shop. This caused him persistent headaches. He got rid of these by moving out and he even survived living rough for one night. He then moved

into a hostel but this wasn't the right place for him so he found his own place to live and is planning to move to an even better flat. He did this through sheer determination, by taking the opportunity to talk things over with his support worker at the hostel, and by focusing on other parts of his body through exercise. All this worked really well for Michael.

2. He handles rejection and hurt by telling himself that it is helpful to know the truth about how people see him. He has also learned to be more independent than his friends and the people he has met in the hostel. He has life skills like being able to cook, look after himself and arrange his finances.

3. He did self-care and relaxation by taking a different approach to de-stressing himself. He stopped looking for a job, got counselling, took more leisure time (exercising sensibly, going on the internet, watching television, and having good coffee), rested more, and started reflecting on things. He is taking things a step at a time. All these things have helped Michael be a lot less stressed.

4. Michael's competent self has a good personality, is popular and daring. He is also intelligent (he did well at school), coordinated (he never fell off his motor bike even though he did some crazy things on it), and he had no jealousy of other people because he felt happy with himself. He is also incredibly brave – he has endured more than most young men of his age.

Tasks to be done

1. More of the same – it is working well. Michael could, perhaps, extend his self-care to sleeping and see if he can improve this too.

2. If he has a better idea of his own, he will do this as well.

Afterthoughts

Steve did think afterwards that maybe Michael could use his reflecting skills to think more about how resentment affects him. This seemed complicated when he tried to explain it but it may turn out to be as much to do with not wanting to hurt other people as well as being balanced. Either way, Steve and Michael can talk more about this next time.

It can be useful to consider sharing information contained in any referral form about the person as this can provide good material for thinking about solutions. Referrals made by professionals are regularly couched in language and concepts that tend to pathologise people, such as 'he is depressive', 'she is enuretic', 'he is frail elderly' or 'she has an attachment disorder'. People can come to believe that *they are the problem* when faced with this, so a solution focused approach would try to encourage detail to begin to question the label.

One way of doing this is to ask people how they 'do' the label, which allows people to explore exceptions to the narrow story being told about them. For example, you may wish to ask someone how they 'do' depression: 'What form does it take?' or 'When is it less of a problem?' or 'Can the depression be scaled?' and 'Is it different at times?' – all of these are questions designed to undermine the label and to develop detail that helps understand how that individual person experiences the problem. Asking people to explain their understanding of problems can help; for example, 'It says here that you have a problem with authority – what does this mean?' or 'You've been diagnosed with autism – how did you get this label?' People are invited to see the problem as the problem, rather than being the problem, and that the worker and the person are there to work together against the problem.

PRACTICE ACTIVITY

Choose a person with whom you are working who has a diagnosis and ask them how useful that diagnosis is to them. What are the advantages of it? What are the disadvantages? Does it help to describe them better? If they could choose their own label, what would it be?

Homework tasks

The previous chapters have provided the opportunity to consider the various techniques that help to develop clear goals, and we find that opening conversations with a 'What needs to happen to make this meeting worth your time and effort?' type of question focuses people on a preferred future. This can take various forms depending on the circumstances and the person, so perhaps, 'If you are able to go home after this meeting and tell your partner that it was really, really helpful, what would have happened?' might be appropriate. Part of being helpful is making sure that the conversation is what people want to talk about, as there can be a temptation to talk about what the professional wants.

Solution focused work commonly includes agreeing tasks in-between the direct face-to-face sessions, which is different from some approaches that presume the worker is needed to advise, guide and lead the person through their difficulties. Following the principles that people are experts in their own lives, that they have strengths and that they can come up with the solution that is most likely to work, we often discuss what tasks are reasonable for them to achieve that will strengthen solutions. This process recognises that they have the capability to take charge of their lives and develop their own resources to sustain a problem-free future. The tasks will, of course, vary from person to person, linked to the identified strengths and exceptions to the specific problems.

CASE EXAMPLE

Avril had an eating problem that she would like to deal with. She had many other problems, including violence when she was a little girl, difficult family dynamics, trouble with sleeping and anxiety and mild epilepsy, but she was keen to focus on her eating as this was important for her now. Avril set a goal of wanting to put on five kilogrammes in the next four months, which would be a healthy weight for her height.

Following her first solution focused session, Avril and her mother came up with several tasks, including: eating a whole meal with the family one day a week; changing her diet to having more cheese and fibre; allowing her mother to cook most of the meals (she is a good cook) but preparing a simple meal on some days for herself; her mother to ask Avril what she wants for dinner and without making a fuss; Avril will tell her mother what she had for lunch without being asked; having a takeaway meal treat once a week; and doing fun activities as a family like they used to do.

The case example demonstrates how helpful tasks can be agreed by everyone concerned based on their understanding of Avril's problem and solutions. The focus on eating actually includes broader work around family dynamics and relationships, so focusing on one problem does not necessarily mean that the others are ignored.

There are different types of homework tasks and we outline just some of them below.

Observational tasks

These help people notice when there are exceptions to the problem or when they have strengths that they hadn't previously seen. In the case example above, Avril may decide to notice what she was doing differently when she was eating a normal meal or when the family was getting on well. People can be asked to recognise what strengths they have that enabled them to achieve their task.

Recognition tasks

Finding ways to assist people to break down the often negative view that they have of themselves is helpful, as is encouraging people to recognise that they can and do have strengths and qualities that can be used to defeat the problem. For example, asking people to make a list of the 20 things that are good about them and bring it to the next meeting can be quite a challenge for some people, so we can encourage this by suggesting that they interview people who know them to find out what they think they are good at. Where one young person struggled to think of anyone who would say good things about him (he had behaved badly, hurt people and his family was very rejecting), we suggested that he interview the family dog to see what good qualities it would say he had. He was able to come to the next meeting with qualities that included being nice to the dog, feeding and caring for it, taking it for regular walks and praising it when it behaved well. The very negative image he had of himself began to dissolve and he was able to see that he had value, which increased his motivation to change.

Pretend tasks

We are particularly fond of pretend tasks as they can be fun as well as productive. Asking someone to pretend when the problem is less of a problem and act accordingly provides opportunities to imagine a problem-free future and what is happening then, providing clues for solutions. And, of course, pretending is almost the same as doing; for example, asking people to notice if others can spot when they are pretending to be confident is always interesting, as it demonstrates that they can be confident and this is validated by others. It also reveals that no one can tell the difference between fake and real confidence.

CASE EXAMPLE

Carol was referred for her aggressive behaviour towards colleagues. She had spent several months with a psychotherapist and had talked at length about her childhood anxieties and her troubled relationship with her controlling father and emotionally distant mother. She did not find this helpful, however, and wanted to focus on her continuing temper problems, so she ended the therapy. The psychotherapist suggested that Carol had unresolved attachment problems that she was resisting and was in need of longer-term intervention.

Carol came to a solution focused worker where she was clear that she wanted to manage her temper, and she could identify exceptions when she was able to do so. She felt that she had 5 control over her behaviour and could see ways to increase that control to 6 by pretending to be 'professional' at times when she felt anger. She planned to pretend to do this over the next week to see who would notice this difference.

When she returned, she was able to recount that people treated her respectfully when she was pretending to be professional, were more inclusive of her and that she did not feel the same levels of anger. She decided that she could easily pretend to be professional more often as this was a better feeling than her previous angry states.

Prediction tasks

There is ample evidence that, generally, we view the successes of others as being due to their personal qualities and our own successes as due to luck ('it just happened'). This makes it difficult for people to recognise exceptions to problems, even when they are clearly happening. When people feel that their problem is out of control, asking them to complete a 'prediction chart' can be helpful. For example, Tom had been diagnosed with ADHD at an early age and, despite significant medication for many years, still found that aged 25 his behaviour was problematic for himself and others, with outbursts of energy and temper. Recently, he was re-diagnosed with adult ADHD. Tom was asked to keep a chart predicting which were going to be good days and which were bad. Once he had achieved some success in his predictions (and there is always some difference that makes a difference), he was able to have a discussion about what was happening differently on those days when things were better. This was in itself useful in thinking about exceptions and strengths, and Tom was able to recognise that he did have some understanding of his situation because even when he predicted a 'bad' day, he was demonstrating that his behaviour was predictable and therefore he had some level of control.

Doing something different

Insanity is often defined as doing the same thing over and over again and expecting different results. It is a common refrain in solution focused work that 'if it isn't working, then do something different', although this can be hard to achieve. Trying something new is part of this, but it can also be about remembering what used to work and bringing this to help with the current situation. Circumstances can make people forget that they have previously dealt with problems in an effective way so encouraging people to think about times they have done this is helpful. Sometimes, people can't think of anything that could be different, especially where they have a long-term physical illness. Here, they can be asked to take one small step in a direction that is good for them, take their time over deciding what this will be, and then tell us about what they decided and how it worked out.

Doing more of the same

If someone reports that they have been making good progress on their problem, then we can only encourage them to develop this further and do more of it. Once people have found their preferred ways of implementing their solutions, the worker can reinforce this by asking more detailed questions about how this was done so that there is a more conscious and nuanced understanding of the strategies. Scales can be used to maintain momentum, so asking people to rate their progress can be useful: 'If 1 is the problem when we first spoke and

10 is the problem completely solved, where are you today? If next time you are able to rate yourself 1 point higher, what needs to happen between now and then?' And doing more of the same is useful when people report that things are not going as well as previously: 'So, what have you forgotten to do that was working for you before?'

Further sessions: What is better?

When someone has a subsequent session, the key question to ask is, 'What is better?' and this should drive the conversation. It is to be hoped that the tasks will have been helpful in changing the problem, or the situation may simply have changed. The question is presumptive in that it assumes that something will be better and asks people to think what this is. Berg (1994) and colleagues at the Brief Family Center developed the acronym *EARS* to describe the structure of these sessions: *E*liciting exceptions and strengths; *A*mplifying them; *R*einforcing them; and *S*tarting again. This approach provides a disciplined focus that is a relentless search for material that can be used to develop solutions.

When things are the same

People may say that nothing has changed since the last time, which can be very demoralising for them. If this happens then, working on the presumption that change always happens, the worker can ask detailed questions about the situation, trying to help identify the smallest changes or differences since the last meeting. It may be that the problem was less of a problem on a particular day or time and by asking the person to describe those days, this increases the likelihood of finding exceptions that can then be amplified. If the person persists in saying that nothing has been different, then one approach is to ask how they have managed to prevent it from being worse, as this then opens up the possibility that they are more resilient than they had thought, with strengths that can then be worked with.

Dolan (1998) describes the 'pessimistic question' where the person seems stuck and cannot yet see any change. Sometimes, problems can be very comfortable as they provide reasons for not facing up to issues or being ready to take on appropriate responsibilities, and protect people from failing. The question is, 'All problems have advantages as well as disadvantages. How can you keep the advantages but still get rid of the problem?' This allows people to think through the pros and cons of their problem and begin to formulate other ways of achieving the good aspects.

When things are worse

There are people who have such difficult and complex histories and lives that they can experience a deterioration of their situation. This may be because of previous problems or it could be that something else has come along and hurt them. As 'life is just one damned thing after another', we cannot expect things to go well all the time, and sometimes this can be dreadful. Using Dolan's 'pessimistic question' can be useful, and avoiding being too optimistic by listening closely to people and talking about how hard change can be helps to validate their feelings. As many people have multiple oppressions and have had many blows in their lives, this is a realistic approach. Asking how they have managed to cope so far with the enormity of the problems, how they have managed to keep going when others may have collapsed, and what would be the first tiny hint that things were improving, all help to acknowledge the problems without accepting that they are unchangeable. Ghul (2015, p.101) suggests asking, 'How are you stopping things getting worse than they already are? Are you giving yourself enough credit for how well you are actually doing? Make a list of at least 30 things you are doing well.'

Multi-agency working

It has been increasingly recognised that people can often have complex needs that can involve a large number of different services and professionals. Finding ways to work together across these different boundaries and disciplines to provide the best care possible is challenging. The following case example shows some of the services needed for a not unusual situation.

> Florence is 85 years old and has lived with her 82 year old husband, George, in their two storey house for the past 40 years. Their son, Andy, emigrated to Australia 12 years ago. When Florence was first diagnosed with dementia in 2010, both she and George were put in touch with a dementia care nurse and

were given information on the disease and the available support that could be on offer if it was required. Together, a plan of care was agreed which could be reviewed and amended whenever Florence's or George's needs changed and included the decision that both Florence and George wanted to live at home for as long as possible in the home that they had shared for so long together. The dementia care nurse kept in close contact with the family and was copied in, at the request of Florence and George, to all correspondence to and from their GP, hospital consultants, community psychiatric nurse, diabetic team and practice nurse to save having to keep telling his story and enabling continuity in the care the couple receive. Recently, George found out he has high blood pressure. He has had to attend regular clinic appointments for check-ups on his hypertension. The dementia care nurse was able to arrange a carer to stay with Florence while he attended his appointments.

(Adapted from National Collaboration for
Integrated Care and Support 2013, p.4)

Of course, Florence and George are also likely to have involvement with local authority adult social care and probably housing services, with input from possibly Age Concern with advice about their finances and welfare entitlements. The drive to integrate services is endorsed by various governmental initiatives, and in England there are clear statements about this: 'We need to create a culture of cooperation and coordination between health, social care, public health, other local services and the third sector. Working in silos is no longer acceptable' (National Collaboration for Integrated Care and Support 2013, p.1). This is underpinned by the principle that: 'My care is planned with people who work together to understand me and my carer(s), put me in control, co-ordinate and deliver services to achieve my best outcomes' (National Voices and Think Local Act Personal 2013, p.3).

How we achieve collaboration is, of course, the issue and is still being developed within our services, and there are questions about how the different status, knowledge, understanding and expertise of disparate professionals can be valued and maximised for the benefit of persons. In order to be effective, we need to be able to understand and respect each other's perspectives and to be able to share information appropriately and clearly. Solution focused approaches do give some pointers for how to work well with other professionals in meetings:

- Keeping your, and the person's, goal in mind at all times. When other practitioners are being negative, remind them of this common purpose.

- Reframing situations, looking for hidden positive motivation.

- Always remembering to compliment other professionals and give them credit for progress.

- Making liberal use of tentative language.

- Asking other professionals what expectations they have of you, what a good outcome of your work would look like to them (Berg and Steiner 2003).

- Repeating and summarising the person's strengths and successes periodically during the meeting.

- Summarising and periodically reminding the person of the professional's good intentions.

(Adapted from Milner and Bateman 2011, p.159)

We have found the Solution Focused Reflective Team approach of Harry Norman to be really helpful in developing teamwork through a purposeful activity. This has six stages and lends itself to the supportive sharing of practice ideas and puzzles, providing a safe space for respectful professional discussions:

1. *Preparation.* Encourage all group members to be clear before the meeting what they would like to gain from it.

2. *Presentation.* The first person presents an issue or situation for the group's consideration.

3. *Clarification.* Each member makes sure that they clearly understand the situation that has been presented by asking questions to clarify the matter and to discover and highlight ways in which the presenter is doing better than they think they are, or has resources that are perhaps underplayed.

4. *Affirmation.* Each member feeds back to the presenter what they have been most impressed with in the presentation. The presenter acknowledges this feedback with a simple 'Thank you.'

5. *Reflection.* Members take turns to say one thing at a time about the presentation. This process goes on until everyone feels they have had their say. If they have no comment to make, they say, 'Pass.' The presenter listens silently in this phase. Contributions tend to build on each other in this phase.

6. *Closing.* The presenter says which parts of the reflection were most relevant and helpful, and may say how they intend to use the feedback in setting a goal to be achieved for next time. The meeting continues with the next presenter.

(Adapted from Norman n.d.)

PRACTICE ACTIVITY

Think of the different professionals you work with in your job:

- Scale how well you think you work together for the benefit of the service users.

- What would have to happen differently for you to scale one point higher?

- Scale how well you understand what those colleagues do and how they do it.

- What would you have to do to scale it one point higher?

- Scale how good you are at multi-disciplinary working.

- What skills, knowledge and qualities do you have that rate you at that scale?

- What would you have to do to scale it one point higher?

Key points

- Change can happen outside the conversations we have with people – look for it and encourage it as it empowers the person to see that they can do it for themselves.

- Use the words of the person as unfiltered as possible – if you begin to interpret, then you are bringing your own expert knowledge to bear, not that of the person.

- Take every opportunity to look for and accentuate strengths and exceptions that will help build solutions – this requires focus, discipline and really listening to the person.

- Some people have terrible lives – they need to be treated with compassion and respect and sensitively encouraged to see a different future.

- It is important to respect other professionals, disciplines and ways of understanding the world – even when they may not respect yours!

References

Allgood, S.M., Parham, K.B., Salts, C.J. and Smith, T.A. (1995) 'The association between pretreatment change and unplanned termination in family therapy.' *American Journal of Family Therapy 23*, 3, 195–202.

Avery, A., Langley-Evans, S.C., Harrington, M. and Swift, J.A. (2016) 'Setting targets leads to greater long-term weight losses and "unrealistic" targets increase the effect in a large community-based commercial weight management group.' *Journal of Human Nutrition and Dietetics 29*, 6, 687–696.

Baker, C. (2015) *Developing Excellent Care for People Living with Dementia in Care Homes.* London: Jessica Kingsley Publishers.

Banat, D., Summers, P. and Pring, T. (2002) 'An investigation into carers' perceptions of the verbal comprehension ability of adults with severe learning disability.' *British Journal of Learning Disabilities 30*, 2, 78–81.

Bannink, F. (2010) *1001 Solution-Focused Questions.* London: W.W. Norton.

Beresford, P. (2007) 'Disability rights and wrongs'. *Disability and Society*, 22, 2, 217–224.

Berg, I.K. (1994) *Family-based Services: A Solution focused approach.* New York, NY: Norton.

Berg, I.K. and Reuss, N.H. (1998) *Solutions Step by Step: A Substance Abuse Treatment Manual.* New York: W.W. Norton.

Berg, I.K. and Steiner, T. (2003) *Children's Solution Work.* London: W.W. Norton.

Bliss, E.V. (2012) 'Solution Focused Brief Therapy.' In R. Raghavan (ed.) *Anxiety and Depression in People with Intellectual Disabilities: Intervention Approaches.* Eynsham: Pavilion Professional.

Bliss, E.V. and Edmonds, G. (2007) *A Self-Determined Future with Asperger Syndrome: Solution Focused Approaches.* London: Jessica Kingsley Publishers.

Boucher, M. (2003) 'Exploring the meaning of tattoos.' *International Journal of Narrative Therapy and Community Work 3*, 57–59.

Bowles, N., Mackintosh, C. and Torn, A. (2001) 'Nurses' communication skills: An evaluation of the impact of solution focused communication training.' *Journal of Advanced Nursing 36*, 3, 347–354.

Bray, D. and Groves, K. (2007) 'A tailor-made psychological approach to palliative care.' *European Journal of Palliative Care 14*, 4, 141–143.

Brindle, N., Branton, T., Stansfield, A. and Zigmond, T. (2013) *A Clinician's Brief Guide to the Mental Capacity Act.* London: RCPsych Publications.

Brown, I. and Brown, R.I. (2003) *Quality of Life and Disability.* London: Jessica Kingsley Publishers.

Bullimore, P. (2003) 'Altering the balance of power: Working with voices.' *International Journal of Narrative Therapy and Community Work 3*, 22–28.

Burns, K. (2016) *Focus on Solutions: A Health Professional's Guide.* 2nd edn. London: Solution Books.

Care Act (2014) Richmond: The National Archives. Accessed on 23/05/2017 at www.legislation.gov.uk/ukpga/2014/23/contents/enacted.

Carr, S.M., Smith, I.C. and Simm, R. (2014) 'Solution-focused brief therapy from the perspective of clients with long-term physical health conditions.' *Psychology, Health & Medicine 19,* 4, 384–391.

Carter, B. (2007) 'Working It Out Together: Being Solution-Focused in the Way We Nurse with Children and Their Families.' In M. McAllister (ed.) *Solution Focused Nursing: Rethinking Practice.* Basingstoke: Palgrave Macmillan.

Costello, B. (2009) 'Kate Moss: The waif that roared: Kate Moss discusses her personal style.' *WWD,* 13 November 2009. Accessed on 24/06/2017 at http://wwd.com/beauty-industry-news/beauty-features/kate-moss-the-waif-that-roared-2367932/

Couzens, A. (1999) 'Sharing the Load: Group Conversations with Young Indigenous Men.' In Dulwich Centre Publications (ed.) *Extending Narrative Therapy: A Collection of Practice-Based Papers.* Adelaide: Dulwich Centre Publications.

Craggs-Hinton, C. (2015) *How to Beat Pain.* London: Sheldon Press.

Crawley, E.M., Gaunt, D.M., Garfield, K. et al.(2017) 'Clinical and cost-effectiveness of the Lightning Process in addition to specialist medical care for paediatric chronic fatigue syndrome: Randomised controlled trial.' *Archives of Disease in Childhood.* Published Online First: 20 September 2017. Doi: 10.1136/archdischild-2017-313375.

Cui, Y., Ke, Z., Li, M., Li, W. and Jiang, L. (2008) 'Application of solution focused model on health education of patients with type 2 diabetes mellitus.' *Journal of PLA Nursing 16,* 20–22.

Dargan, P.J., Simm, R. and Murray, C. (2014) 'New approaches towards chronic pain: Patient experiences of a solution focused pain management programme.' *British Journal of Pain 8,* 1, 34–42.

De Jong, P. and Berg, I.K. (2008) *Interviewing for Solutions.* 3rd edn. Pacific Grove, CA: Brooks/Cole.

De Shazer, S. (1988) *Clues: Investigating Solutions in Brief Therapy.* New York: W.W. Norton.

De Shazer, S. (1991) *Putting Difference to Work.* New York: W.W. Norton.

De Shazer, S. (1994) *Words Were Originally Magic.* New York: W.W. Norton.

De Valda, M. (2003) 'From paranoid schizophrenia to hearing voices – and other class distinctions.' *International Journal of Narrative Therapy and Community Work 3,* 13–17.

Denmark, J.C. (1994) *Deafness and Mental Health.* London: Jessica Kingsley Publishers.

Dennison, L., Moss-Morris, R. and Chalder, T. (2009) 'A review of psychological correlates of adjustment in patients with multiple sclerosis.' *Clinical Psychology Review 29,* 141–153.

Department for Children, Schools and Families (2008) *2020 Children and Young People's Workforce Strategy.* DCSF Publications, Nottingham.

Department of Health (2004) *Mental Health Policy Implementation Guide.* London: HMSO.

Department of Health (2005) National Service Framework for Long-Term Conditions. London: HMSO.

Department of Health (2007) *Independence, Choice and Risk: A Guide to Best Practice in Supported Decision Making.* London: HMSO.

Department of Health (2011) *Statement of Government Policy on Adult Safeguarding.* London: HMSO. Accessed on 23/05/2017 at https://www.gov.uk/government/uploads/system/uploads/attachment_data/file/215591/dh_126770.pdf.

Dolan, Y. (1998) *One Small Step: Moving beyond Trauma and Therapy to a Life of Joy.* Watsonville, CA: Papier-Mache Press.

Edwards, L.M. and Pedrotti, J.T. (2004) 'Utilizing the strengths of our cultures: Therapy with biracial women and girls.' *Women and Therapy 27*, 1&2, 33–43.

Elgin, S. (2000) *The Language Imperative.* Cambridge, MA: Perseus Books.

Epston, D. (1998) *Catching Up with David Epston: A Collection of Narrative Practice-Based Papers, 1991–1996.* Adelaide: Dulwich Centre Publications.

Forshaw, M. (2002) *Essential Health Psychology.* London: Arnold.

Freeman, J., Epston, D. and Lobovits, D. (1997) *Playful Approaches to Serious Problems: Narrative Therapy with Children and Their Families.* New York: W.W. Norton.

Furman, B. and Ahola, T. (1992) *Solution Talk.* New York: W.W. Norton.

Gallop, R. and Stamina, E. (2003) 'The person who is suicidal.' In P. Barker (ed.) *Psychiatric and Mental Health Nursing: The Craft of Caring.* Oxford: Oxford University Press.

Gallop, R. and Tully, T. (2003) 'The person who self-harms.' In P. Barker (ed.) *Psychiatric and Mental Health Nursing: The Craft of Caring.* Oxford: Oxford University Press.

Ghul, R. (2015) *The Power of the Next Small Step.* Keller, TX: The Connie Institute.

Goldsmith, S. (2015a) 'Getting the "Fundamentals" Right.' In C. Baker *Developing Excellent Care for People Living with Dementia in Care Homes.* London: Jessica Kingsley Publishers.

Goldsmith, S. (2015b) 'Proactive Analysis and Follow-through.' in C. Baker *Developing Excellent Care for People Living with Dementia in Care Homes.* London: Jessica Kingsley Publishers.

Goleman, D. (1995) *Emotional Intelligence.* New York: Bantam.

Grey, C. (2010) *The New Social Story Book.* Arlington, TX: Future Horizons.

Gridley, K., Brooks, J. and Glendenning, C. (2012) *Good Support for People with Complex Needs: What Does It Look Like and Where is the Evidence? Research Findings.* London: NIHR School for Social Care Research.

Hackett, P. (2005) 'Ever Appreciating Circles.' *Journal of Family Psychotherapy* 16, 1–2, 83–84.

Haines, S. (2015) *Trauma is Really Strange.* London: Jessica Kingsley Publishers.

Hawkes, D., Marsh, T.I. and Wilgosh, R. (1998) *Solution Focused Therapy: A Handbook for Health Care Professionals.* Oxford: Butterworth-Heinemann.

Henden, J. (2008) *Preventing Suicide: The Solution Focused Approach.* Chichester: Wiley.

Howe, D. (2008) *The Emotionally Intelligent Social Worker.* Basingstoke: Palgrave Macmillan.

Iveson, C. (2002) 'Solution-focused Brief Therapy.' *Advances in Psychiatric Treatment 8*, 2, 149–56.

Iveson, C. (1990) *Whose Life? Community Care of Older People and Their Families.* London: Brief Therapy Press.

Iveson, C. (2002) *Whose Life? Community Care of Older People and Their Families.* 2nd edn. London: BT Press.

Jacob, F. (2001) *Solution-Focused Recovery from Eating Distress.* London: BT Press.

Johnson, L.N., Nelson, T.S. and Allgood, S.M. (1998) 'Noticing pretreatment change and therapeutic outcome: An initial study.' *American Journal of Family Therapy 26*, 2, 159–168.

Jones, V. and Northway, R. (2006) 'Children with Learning Disabilities.' In A. Glasper and J. Richardson (eds) *A Textbook of Children's and Young People's Nursing.* Edinburgh: Churchill Livingstone.

Kerr, D. (2007) *Understanding Learning Disability and Dementia: Developing Effective Interventions.* London: Jessica Kingsley Publishers.

Lahad, M., Shacham, M. and Ayalon, O. (2012) *The 'BASIC Ph' Model of Coping and Resiliency.* London: Jessica Kingsley Publishers.

Lewycka, M. (2002) *Caring for Someone with a Sight Problem.* London: Age Concern.

Licence, K. (2005) 'Promoting a healthy diet and physical activity for children and young people – the evidence.' in R. Chambers and K. Licence (eds) *Looking After Children in Primary Care: A Companion to the Children's National Service Framework*. Abingdon: Radcliffe Publishing.

Lloyd, H.F., Macdonald, A. and Wilson, L. (2016) 'Solution-Focused Brief Therapy.' In N. Beail (ed.) *Psychological Therapies for People Who Have Intellectual Disabilities*. Leicester: British Psychological Society.

Lulé, D., Zickler, C., Häcker, S., Bruno, M.A., Demertzi, A., Pellas, F. and Kübler, A. (2009) 'Life can be worth living in locked-in syndrome.' *Progress in Brain Research 177*, 339–351.

McAllister, M. (2007) 'The Spirit of SFN: Making Change at Three Levels.' In M. McAllister (ed.) *Solution Focused Nursing: Rethinking Practice*. Basingstoke: Palgrave Macmillan.

Macdonald, A. (2010) 'The impact of the Mental Capacity Act on social workers' decision-making and the assessment of risk.' *British Journal of Social Work 40*, 1229–1246.

Macdonald, A. (2011) *Solution-Focused Therapy: Theory, Research and Practice*. 2nd edn. London: Sage.

MacKinlay, E. and Trevitt, C. (2012) *Finding Meaning in the Expression of Dementia*. London: Jessica Kingsley Publishers.

Marriott, H. (2003) *The Selfish Pig's Guide to Caring*. London: Sphere Books.

Marsh, R. and Hudson, J. (2014) *Locked In: One Man's Miraculous Escape from the Terrifying Confines of Locked-In Syndrome*. London: Piatkus.

Mattelin, E. and Volckaert, H. (2017) *Autism and Solution-Focused Practice*. London: Jessica Kingsley Publishers.

Mayer, J.D., Salovey, P. and Caruso, D.R. (2004) 'Emotional Intelligence: theory, findings, and implications'. *Psychological inquiry 15,3*, 197–215.

Mencap (2007) *Death by* Indifference: *Following Up the* Treat Me Right! *Report*. London: Mencap. Accessed on 23/05/2017 at https://www.mencap.org.uk/sites/default/files/2016-06/DBIreport.pdf.

Michael, J. and Richardson, A. (2008) 'Healthcare for all: The independent inquiry into access to healthcare for people with learning disabilities.' *Tizard Learning Disability Review 13*, 4, 28–34.

Miller, G. (1997) *Becoming Miracle Workers: Language and Meaning in Brief Therapy*. New York: Aldine de Gruyter.

Milner, J. (2001) *Women and Social Work: Narrative Approaches*. Basingstoke: Palgrave Macmillan.

Milner, J. (2004) 'Groupwork with young women.' *Context 74*, 14–17.

Milner, J. (2008a) 'Don't Tell Me How I Should Feel about My Breast Cancer.' *Daily Telegraph*, 6 October, 2008.

Milner, J. (2008b) 'Solution-focused approaches to caring for children whose behaviour is sexually harmful.' *Adoption and Fostering 32*, 42–50.

Milner, J. and Bateman, J. (2011) *Working with Children and Teenagers Using Solution Focused Practice: Enabling Children to Overcome Challenges and Achieve their Potential*. London: Jessica Kingsley Publishers.

Milner, J. and Myers, S. (2016) *Working with Violence and Confrontation Using Solution Focused Approaches*. London: Jessica Kingsley Publishers.

Milner, J. and Myers, S. (2017) *Creative Ideas for Solution Focused Practice: Inspiring Guidance, Ideas and Activities*. London: Jessica Kingsley Publishers.

Milner, J., Myers, S. and O'Byrne, P. (2015) *Assessment in Social Work*. 4th edn. Basingstoke: Palgrave Macmillan.

Milner, J. and O'Byrne, P. (2002a) *Assessment in Social Work.* 2nd edn. Basingstoke: Palgrave Macmillan.

Milner, J. and O'Byrne, P. (2002b) *Brief Counselling: Narratives and Solutions.* Basingstoke: Palgrave Macmillan.

Milner, J. and O'Byrne, P. (2004) *Assessment in Counselling: Theory, Process and Decision Making.* Basingstoke: Palgrave Macmillan.

Mishima, N. (2012) 'Applying a Solution-Focused Approach to Health Interviews in Japan.' In C. Franklin, T.S. Trepper, W.J. Gingerich and E.E. McCollum (eds) *Solution-Focused Brief Therapy: A Handbook of Evidence-Based Practice.* New York: Oxford University Press.

Murray Parkes, C. (1986) *Bereavement: Studies of Grief in Adult Life.* New edn. Harmondsworth: Penguin.

Musker, M. (2007) 'Learning Disabilities and Solution Focused-Nursing.' In M. MacAllister (ed.) *Solution Focused Nursing: Rethinking Practice.* Basingstoke: Palgrave Macmillan.

Myers, S. and Milner, J. (2007) *Sexual Issues in Social Work.* Bristol: Policy Press.

National Collaboration for Integrated Care and Support (2013) *Integrated Care and Support: Our Shared Commitment.* London: National Collaboration for Integrated Care and Support. Accessed on 23/05/2017 at www.gov.uk/government/uploads/system/uploads/attachment_data/file/198748/DEFINITIVE_FINAL_VERSION_Integrated_Care_and_Support_-_Our_Shared_Commitment_2013-05-13.pdf.

National Voices and Think Local Act Personal (2013) *A Narrative for Person-Centred Coordinated Care.* London: NHS England. Accessed on 23/05/2017 at www.england.nhs.uk/wp-content/uploads/2013/05/nv-narrative-cc.pdf.

Nelson-Becker, H., Chapin, R. and Fast, B. (2013) 'The Strengths Model with Older Adults: Critical Practice Components.' In D. Saleebey (ed.) *The Strengths Perspective in Social Work Practice.* International 6th edn. Boston, MA: Pearson Education.

NICE (2009) *Depression: The Treatment and Management of Depression in Adults.* NICE clinical guideline 90. London: National Institute for Health and Clinical Excellence.

NICE (2011) *Alcohol-Use Disorders: Diagnosis, Assessment and Management of Harmful Drinking and Alcohol Dependence.* NICE Clinical guideline 115. London: National Institute for Health and Clinical Excellence.

Norlander, L. and McSteen, K. (2001) *Choices at the End of Life: Finding out What Your Parents Want before It's Too Late.* Minneapolis, MN: Fairview Press.

Norman, H. (n.d.) *Solution Focused Reflecting Teams.* Bristol: Harry Norman Partnership. Accessed on 23/05/2017 at http://sfwork.com/solworld/downloads/SFRTeamPrimer02.pdf.

Panayotov, P.A., Strahilov, B.E. and Anichkina, A.Y. (2012) 'Solution-Focused Brief Therapy and Medication Adherence with Schizophrenic Patients.' In C. Franklin, T.S. Trepper, W.J. Gingerich and E.E. McCollum (eds) *Solution-Focused Brief Therapy: A Handbook of Evidence-Based Practice.* New York: Oxford University Press.

Polaschek, L. and Polaschek, N. (2007) 'Solution focused conversations: A new therapeutic strategy in well nursing consultations.' *Journal of Advanced Nursing 59,* 2, 111–119.

Reiter, M.D. (2010) 'Hope and expectancy in solution-focused brief therapy.' *Journal of Family Psychotherapy 21,* 2, 132–148.

Reivich, K. and Shatte, A. (2003) *The Resilience Factor: 7 Key Ways to Finding Your Inner Strength and Overcoming Life's Hurdles.* London: Broadway Books.

Rheingold, H. (1998) *They Have a Word for It: A Lighthearted Lexicon of Untranslatable Words and Phrases.* Los Angeles, CA: Jeremy P. Tarcher.

Roeden, J.M., Bannink, F.P., Maaskant, M.A. and Curfs, L.M.G. (2009) 'Solution-focused brief therapy with persons with intellectual difficulties.' *Journal of Policy and Practise in Intellectual Disabilities 6*, 4, 253–259.

Rogers, C.R. (1951) Client-Centred Therapy. London: Constable.

Rogers, C.R. (19610 on Being a person. Boston: Houghton Mifflin.

Rogers, C.R. (1980) A Way of Being Boston: Houghton Mifflin.

Ross, M. (1996) 'Learning to Listen to Children.' In R. Davie, G. Upton and V. Varma (eds) *The Voice of the Child: A Handbook for Professionals*. London: Falmer Press.

Rycroft, C., Gorer, G., Storr, A., Wren-Lewis, J. and Lomas, P. (eds) (1966) *Psychoanalysis Observed*. Harmondsworth: Penguin.

Saleebey, D. (ed.) (2013) *The Strengths Perspective in Social Work Practice*. International 6th edn. Boston, MA: Pearson Education.

Scragg, T. (2012) 'Working with Loss and Bereavement in Older People.' In B. Hall and T. Scragg (eds) *Social Work with Older People*. Maidenhead: Open University Press.

Selekman, M.D. (1997) *Pathways to Change: Brief Therapy Solutions with Difficult Adolescents*. New York: Guilford Press.

Selekman, M.D. (2002) *Living on the Razor's Edge*. New York: W.W. Norton.

Selekman, M.D. (2007) *The Optimistic Child: A Proven Program to Safeguard Children against Depression and Building Lifelong Resilience*. New York: Houghton Mifflin.

Sharry, J. (2011) *Becoming a Solution Detective*. 2nd edn. London: Routledge.

Sharry, J., Madden, B. and Darmody, M. (2001) *Becoming a Solution Focused Detective: A Strengths-Based Guide to Brief Therapy*. London: BT Press.

Shone, N. (2013) *Coping Successfully with Chronic Illness*. London: Sheldon Press.

Simm, R., Iddon, J. and Barker, C. (2014) 'A community pain service solution-focused pain management programme: Delivery and preliminary outcome data.' *British Journal of Pain 8*, 1, 49–56.

Social Services and Well-being (Wales) Act (2014) Accessed on 23/05/2017 at http:// gov.wales/docs/dhss/publications/160127socialservicesacten.pdf.

Staton, J., Shuy, R. and Byrock, I. (2001) *A Few Months to Live: Different Paths to Life's End*. Washington, DC: Georgetown University Press.

Stern, D. (2011) 'Narrative therapy at any age.' *International Journal of Narrative Therapy and Community Work 1*, 57–64.

Swaffer, K. (2016) *What the Hell Happened to My Brain? Living beyond Dementia*. London: Jessica Kingsley Publishers.

Talmon, M. (1990) *Single Session Therapy: Maximizing the Effect of the First (and often only) Therapeutic Encounter*. San Francisco, CA: Jossey – Bass.

Thompson, N. (2003) *Communication and Language: A Handbook of Theory and Practice*. Basingstoke: Macmillan.

Timmins, S. (forthcoming) *Developing Resilience in Young People with Autism Using Social Stories*. London: Jessica Kingsley Publishers.

Tizard, B. and Clarke, A. (eds) (2000) *Vulnerability and Resilience in Human Development*. London: Jessica Kingsley Publishers.

Turnell, A. and Edwards, S. (1999) *Signs of Safety: A Solution and Safety Oriented Approach to Child Protection Casework*. New York: W.W. Norton.

Turnell, A. and Essex, S. (2006) *Working with 'Denied' Child Abuse: The Resolutions Approach*. Maidenhead: Open University Press.

Unwin, D. (2005) 'SFGP! Why a solution focused approach is brilliant in primary care.' *Solution News 1*, 10–12.

Walsh, K. and Moss, C. (2007) 'Solution Focused Mental Health Nursing.' In M. McAllister (ed.) *Solution Focused Nursing: Rethinking Practice*. Basingstoke: Palgrave Macmillan.

Walsh, T. (2010) *The Solution Focused Helper: Ethics and Practice in Health and Social Care.* Maidenhead: McGraw Hill and Oxford University Press.

White, C. (2001) 'Cognitive behavioral principles in managing chronic disease.' *Western Journal of Medicine 175*, 5, 338–342.

White, M. (1995) *Re-authoring Lives: Interviews and Essays.* Adelaide: Dulwich Centre Publications.

White, M. and Epston, D. (1990) *Narrative Means to Therapeutic Ends.* New York: W.W. Norton.

White, N. and Bateman, J. (2008) 'The use of narrative therapy to allow the emergence of engagement.' *International Journal of Narrative Therapy and Community Work 2*, 17–28.

Whiting, L. (2006) 'Children and Their Families.' In I. Peate and L. Whiting (eds) *Caring for Children and their Families.* Chichester: Wiley.

Williams, J. (2003) 'The use of humour and other coping strategies.' *International Journal of Narrative Therapy and Community Work 3*, 5–8.

Winbolt, B. (2011) *Solution Focused Therapy for the Helping Professions.* London: Jessica Kingsley Publishers.

Wittgenstein, L. (1963) *Philosophical Investigations.* 3rd edn. Oxford: Blackwell.

Wittgenstein, L. (1980) *Remarks on the Philosophy of Psychology.* Oxford: Blackwell.

Subject Index

Author Index